Adult Hydrothe

D1504440

DATE DUE

Long have the praises of water been sung. It has cleansed cult and creed, cured pysche and soma.
Christa and Jost Benedum

And grew a seething bath which yet men prove, against strange maladies a sovereign cure.
Shakespeare

Adult Hydrotherapy
A practical approach

Edited by

Margaret Reid Campion
Grad.Dip Physiotherapy (UK) MCSP, MAPA
Curtin University of Technology, Western Australia

Foreword by
Professor Lance Twomey
Professor and Head of School of Physiotherapy,
Curtin University of Technology, Western Australia

Heinemann Medical Books

To all our patients who have taught us all so much as they tolerated our ministrations

Heinemann Medical Books
An imprint of Heinemann Professional Publishing
Halley Court, Jordan Hill, Oxford OX2 8EJ

OXFORD   LONDON   SINGAPORE   NAIROBI   IBADAN   KINGSTON

First published 1990

British Library Cataloguing in Publication Data
Adult hydrotherapy
  1. Medicine. Hydrotherapy
  I. Campion, Margaret Reid
  615. 853

ISBN 0 433 00088 0

Typeset by Latimer Trend Ltd, Plymouth and printed in
Great Britain by Biddles Ltd, Guildford and Kings Lynn

Contents

Foreword by *Professor Lance Twomey*   vi

Preface   viii

Acknowledgements   x

List of Contributors   xii

Section I   Hydrotherapy—an overview   1
  1   Introduction to hydrotherapy   *M. Reid Campion*   3
  2   Techniques of exercise in water and therapeutic
      swimming   *M. Reid Campion*   21

Section II   Hydrotherapy—a means of rehabilitation   39
  3   Hydrotherapy for the neuro-surgical patient
      G. 'Jega' Jegasothy   41
  4   Hydrotherapy in neurological rehabilitation
      K. Smith   70
  5   Hydrotherapy in spinal cord injuries   *J. McGibbon
      and W. Elford*   104
  6   Hydrotherapy in rheumatic disease and fibrositis
      L. M. Tinsley and B. Laing   123
  7   Hydrotherapy in orthopaedics   *K. Blades*   156
  8   Hydrotherapy for sports injuries   *D. Hopper*   177

Section III   Health promotion   199
  9   Hydrotherapy in the childbearing year   *C. Dyson*   201
 10   Aqua relaxation for mothers and babies   *R. Mori*   226
 11   Water fitness for the older adult   *M. Skreiner*   238

Index   248

Foreword

Exercise in water is an essential part of physiotherapy and has to be considered as a serious option in the physical rehabilitation of persons of all ages. Water provides a superb medium for exercise, since it offers opportunity for treatment which is not available within traditional land-based exercise programmes. It is an excellent means of providing therapy since most patients enjoy their time in the water, find it supportive and comfortable and great fun. Hydrotherapy allows even the most fragile patient the opportunity of purposeful movement and can serve as the starting point for a graduated comprehensive exercise regimen leading the individual into a more active rewarding lifestyle. On the other hand, it may also be used for the fit strong sports competitor as an important part of the rehabilitation process after injury, leading back to full sports participation.

Margaret Reid Campion is internationally known as a leader and innovator in hydrotherapy. She is constantly involved in advising on therapeutic management in water, assisting with pool design and as a teacher of hydrotherapy skills. She has pioneered the 'Halliwick' approach to exercises in water in the southern hemisphere and is truly a world leader in this important therapeutic area. During her time in Western Australia, her enthusiasm has attracted a large complement of physiotherapists who have further developed and applied hydrotherapy skills to the treatment of a variety of neuro-musculoskeletal disorders. It has been pleasing to see the extraordinary development of hydrotherapy in Western Australia and the enthusiasm with which physiotherapists are re-discovering their interest in this age-old therapy modality.

This book *Adult Hydrotherapy: a Practical Approach* is a most important complement to Mrs Reid Campion's previous publication *Hydrotherapy in Paediatrics* (Heinemann Medical Books, 1985) which has been so well accepted. In this instance, she has been joined by nine superb clinicians to bring a range of expertise to the treatment of adults. The Western Australian lifestyle centres on outdoor life and water sports and, in this context, it is not surprising to see scholarly applied text and reference books on hydrotherapy originate. It must be stressed that this is a text which concentrates on the practical issues involved in rehabilitation and fitness and will be used as an important reference for those interested in effective treatment.

Lance Twomey, PhD
Professor and Head of School of Physiotherapy
Curtin University of Technology

Preface

This book is the result of the cooperation and liaison between a number of physiotherapists in Western Australia.

For some years they have been treating a wide variety of patients in the hydrotherapy pool. Each of the physiotherapists is a specialist in his or her field treating their patients on land as well as in the water. This situation provides a unique and enviable experience and gives these physiotherapists the opportunity to observe their patients on land and in the water where different forces apply and techniques of treatment vary. The presence of buoyancy in water in addition to gravity provides the possibility of other dimensions for exercise.

In water the hydrodynamical principles of buoyancy, metacentre and the rotational effects, provide opportunities for specialized techniques. Turbulence is a further factor, for whilst occurring in air it is hardly felt, however, in water every movement produces turbulence which can be appreciated by the human being. The weight of water means that it can be leant against and thus a force is provided against which the individual can work.

Early treatment in a weight relieving situation is possible and the warmth and support of the water provide other beneficial effects. A greater perception of rotational effects with the need to control these, gives rise to techniques which demand considerable balance and coordination as well as precise muscle work.

The contributors have provided a practical guide to hydrotherapy for a variety of conditions. All agreed that to offer total recipes was not appropriate. They trust that in writing their chapters they have supplied useful suggestions which will help physiotherapists to commence the treatment of many different diseases and disabilities. At the same time, it is the contributors' intention to provoke thought about treatment programmes and that physiotherapists will develop lateral thinking in order that the treatment programmes they conduct in water be enhanced. In this way hydrotherapy may be understood and recognized by doctors and physiotherapists as a valuable modality in its own right as part of the total rehabilitation programme for a wide variety of conditions.

For the sake of convenience, the patient is referred to as 'he' and the physiotherapist as 'she'.

Acknowledgements

Following the success of *Hydrotherapy in Paediatrics*, Heinemann Medical Books invited me to write a companion volume for adults. Since some exciting developments were taking place in the field of hydrotherapy in Western Australia it seemed appropriate to invite those physiotherapists most involved in treating patients in their area of speciality, both on land and in the water, to contribute to such a book.

Western Australia was the first state in Australia to establish a Hydrotherapy Special Interest Group—in fact this was almost certainly a world first. In addition, the group established standards for hydrotherapy which were adopted by the Australian Physiotherapy Association—Western Australian Branch. However, it was in the hydrotherapy pool itself that other interesting developments were occurring, ideas flowing and treatments changing.

There were guarded responses when I approached the physiotherapists involved, but all expressed their willingness to try and write about their speciality and hydrotherapy. Since then their enthusiasm has encouraged and helped me in my task as editor and author. I owe all the contributors a deep debt of gratitude.

In writing a part of this book, I have tried to present material that complements hydrotherapy, the work of the other authors and to present some ideas and approaches that reflect the hydrotherapy currently being undertaken and developed in Western Australia. Editing has not been easy, I have refrained from detracting from the essence and personalized writing of the other authors. I am aware that in so doing a lack of uniformity may be criticized, but it seemed important that each chapter should primarily reflect the author and his or her approach to hydrotherapy.

Since a book of this kind is not the work of a few, we would like to thank all who contributed in various ways. Special thanks are due to Wendy Alford who produced the drawings which add to the clarity of actions of the physiotherapists and patients.

All of us would wish to record our gratitude to our many patients over the years who have accepted our ministrations and taught us all so much.

A number of people have typed the various chapters and each author wishes to thank them. My personal thanks are due to each and everyone of them. I wish to record my personal thanks to Michelle Connolly who supported me by typing my contributions to this book as well as other parts of the manuscript.

Professor Lance Twomey who has written the foreword, for which we are all most grateful, has continued to support the efforts of the authors and myself. He recognizes the importance and value of our work in hydrotherapy and supports our efforts through the undergraduate and postgraduate programmes through the School of Physiotherapy at Curtin University of Technology.

Working from the northern to the southern hemisphere and almost halfway round the world can create difficulties but the staff of Heinemann Medical Books have shown great patience and courtesy and offered many helpful suggestions. We thank them all for their consideration and cooperation.

Last but no means least, I would like to record my thanks to all the partners and families of the co-authors who accepted the necessary deprivations as the writers worked to meet the deadline and thus contributed to the book.

Margaret Reid Campion
Editor and Author

Contributors

Kevin Blades, BAppSc (Physio), MAPA

Since qualifying in 1979, Kevin has worked at The Royal Perth Rehabilitation Hospital in areas such as soft tissue injuries, spinal injuries, neurology, amputations and orthopaedics treating both out- and in-patients. Appointed Senior Physiotherapist in Orthopaedics in 1982, Kevin has continued to work in the area with his special interest being hydrotherapy, joint-replacement and continuous passive movement (CPM). He has been Secretary of the Western Australian Hydrotherapy Special Interest Group since its inception in 1984.

Cherry Dyson, BSc Physio (WA), MAPA

Cherry trained in the UK and then worked in South Africa for eight years gaining experience in neurology, cardiology and plastic surgery. Arriving in Western Australia, Cherry was appointed Senior Physiotherapist at Osborne Park Hospital, Perth, and then joined the Parenthood Unit at Community Health Service. Specializing in Obstetrics and Gynaecology Cherry has run Antenatal preparation, healthy pregnancy and postnatal classes as well as assessing and treating individual problems. Antenatal and postnatal classes in water run by Cherry are highly successful.

Wendy Elford, BAppSc (Physio) MAPA

After graduating from W.A.I.T. in 1982, Wendy practised in Perth and overseas before taking up a position at the Royal Perth (Rehabilitation) Hospital in 1985. She has worked extensively in both the acute management and rehabilitation of spinal cord injuries and is currently working as a senior physiotherapist in neurosurgery at the Sir Charles Gairdener Hospital, Perth. She aims to complete a postgraduate diploma in neuroscience in the near future.

Diana Hopper, BAppSc (WAIT), MEd (WA), DipYL (SWDVic), TC, GradDip SPhysio (WAIT), FA, MAPA, FRSMF.

Sport, sports physiotherapy and recreation are strongly represented in Diana's career. Presently a Senior Lecturer, School of Physiotherapy, Curtin University, she has had considerable international experience in Zimbabwe, Kobe Japan, at the World Cup Athletics and is the Australian Physiotherapist for the Australian Rhythmic Gymnastics Group. Diana has held most of the executive positions in the ASMF in the last fifteen years and was awarded a Foundation Fellowship by the Federation in 1985. Her 'passion' is swimming and her ability as a swimmer and swimming coach has led to wide interest and concern in this field of sport.

G. 'Jega' Jegasothy, Associateship Physiotherapy MAPA

'Jega' qualified in 1972 and for four years worked as a physiotherapist in the University Hospital, Kuala Lumpur, Malaysia. Since returning to Western Australia, where she trained, Jega has worked in the Neurosurgical Unit at Royal Perth Rehabilitation Hospital and has been Senior Physiotherapist to the 28 bed ward for eight years. Her hydrotherapy programmes have some very innovative features.

Beverley Laing, DipPty (Vic), MAPA

Bev's professional career has largely centred on rheumatology. Having trained in Melbourne, she worked in Victoria prior to moving to Western Australia in 1979. Her work as travelling physiotherapist for WA Arthritis and Rheumatism Foundation was followed by other posts where rheumatology, hydrotherapy and splinting played major roles. Her abiding interest in this field has led to involvement in research and currently she is clinical metrologist for various rheumatology trials at two major Perth hospitals as well as studying the value of a comprehensive treatment programme for fibrositis patients including hydrotherapy.

Jane McGibbon, BAppSc (WAIT), MAPA

Prior to being appointed to the Special Unit at Royal Perth Rehabilitation Hospital, Jane worked in the Out-patients Department, the Sports Injuries Clinic, the Amputee Clinic and on the Orthopaedic Wards. Apart from treating the spinal injury patients Jane was team physiotherapist to many State and Australian Wheelchair Sport teams. Typically, in a very busy life she held numerous positions in the Australian Physiotherapy Association at both State and National Levels.

Rosalie Mori, BAppSc (Physio), MAPA

After qualifying in 1981 Rosalie worked at Albany Regional Hospital treating orthopaedic out-patients and in-patients, both adults and children. A two year spell at a Special School in Perth followed. Here she treated the physically handicapped pupils at the school as well as children with MCD from the surrounding community.

In March 1984, Rosalie returned to Albany as the Paediatric Physiotherapist. Her work is carried out in the hospital, in homes, schools and in the community in general which means her case load is very diverse.

Margaret Reid Campion, GradDip Physiotherapy (UK), MCSP, MAPA

After years of general work, then paediatrics and hydrotherapy Margaret left England and settled in Western Australia. In 1978, she joined the teaching staff of the School of Physiotherapy as a Lecturer. Travelling and teaching in Australia and many countries overseas in addition to teaching under- and postgraduate students are all part of Margaret's life. Author of *Hydrotherapy in Paediatrics*, she has contributed to Duffield's *Exercise in Water* and written extensively.

Although hydrotherapy and related topics are of especial interest to Margaret she says she has other 'loves' such as obstetrics and gynaecology, paediatrics and neurology.

Margaret Skreiner, DipPty (WA), MAPA

Margaret has both physiotherapy and arts at her finger tips. She has worked as a physiotherapist to the Alcohol and Drug Authority at a Senior Citizens Village and currently for the Western Australian Health Department running fitness programmes for the over 50's including water fitness groups.

Karen Smith, Associateship Physiotherapy, MAPA

Currently Senior Physiotherapist of the Neurology Unit at the Royal Perth Rehabilitation Hospital, Karen has had wide experience in neurology combined with hydrotherapy in London and Montreal. Her abiding interest in neurology has involved her in graduate studies in neuro-sciences and a number of neurological courses including a Bobath course at McGill University, Montreal.

Lynnette Tinsley, DipPty (WA), MAPA

Lyn is currently involved with treatment and patient education of rheumatic diseased patients as well as teaching undergraduate and postgraduate physiotherapists, and other health professionals.

She has worked in varied posts in Western Australia and is presently Senior Physiotherapist to the Rheumatic Diseases Unit at Royal Perth Rehabilitation Hospital. Her overseas experience was gained in London, Norway and Denmark. In 1981 she was awarded a Churchill Fellowship and travelled in the UK and Scandinavia. Ankylosing Spondylosis is an area of special interest to Lyn.

HYDROTHERAPY—AN OVERVIEW

INTRODUCTION TO SECTION I

This section of the book aims to introduce hydrotherapy and many aspects of the modality.

Physiotherapists are today being asked to take an increasing number of patients into the hydrotherapy pool for rehabilitation. This together with the long history of the use of water for both therapeutic and recreational purposes behoves the profession to develop appropriate training at both the undergraduate and the postgraduate levels.

It is essential that the physiotherapist has the fullest understanding of all aspects pertaining to hydrotherapy and therapeutic swimming from the mechanics of fluids to pool design and from physiological effects to modern techniques.

Above all, the uniqueness of water should be used as a resource for rehabilitation in its own right. Assessment, recording and research are vital to the ultimate and appropriate use of the medium in restoring health.

The ensuing chapters attempt to provide a base for hydrotherapeutic knowledge, to explore techniques and to encourage and develop assessment and recording procedures so that, with confidence, the physiotherapist can promote the value of hydrotherapy for many diseases and disabilities.

Introduction to Hydrotherapy

Hydrotherapy as a modality for rehabilitation has a long history and is as important today as it was in the past. With the current upsurge in the popularity of hydrotherapy, physiotherapists are encouraged to use water, making the most of its unique properties. Hydrotherapeutic techniques must be learnt and new ideas explored and developed.

This chapter reviews hydrotherapy in general and sets the scene, as it were, for the ensuing chapters. A brief statement on the historical background precedes notes on hydrodynamical principles. Only those principles with particular relevance to hydrotherapeutic techniques are touched on. The importance of assessment and recording is discussed and a format for each presented.

An attempt is made to rationalize some points such as the temperature at which water should be kept for hydrotherapy, and the teaching of mental adjustment and balance restoration as prerequisites for hydrotherapy. Techniques of exercise are reviewed briefly where these have been extensively explained by other authors (Bolton and Goodwin, 1974; Skinner and Thomson, 1983; Davis and Harrison, 1988). The development of exercise based on hydrodynamical principles which produce movement as a reaction, increase balance and co-ordination and enhance movement is presented. Group work is discussed in general terms and in relation to hydrotherapy sessions that may include both group and individual work.

Swimming has an important role in the maintenance of health and general fitness. Swimming forms part of many rehabilitative water programmes and is usually developed by the physiotherapist, thus therapeutic swimming comes within their province.

HISTORICAL BACKGROUND

By necessity this is a brief review of the use of water for therapeutic purposes throughout the ages. The study of the historical background of both the curative and recreational aspects of water is fascinating. It has been dealt with by a number of authors (Wyman, 1944; Krizek, 1963; Price, 1981) and the interested reader is referred to their work.

The history of hydrotherapy as a modality used in physical medicine goes back many thousands of years. At which moment in time hydrotherapy was first used therapeutically is not known, but records dating back to 2400 BC suggest that Proto-Indian culture made hygienic installations and that the early Egyptians, Assyrians and Mohammedans used mineral waters for curative purposes. The Hindus in 1500 BC, used water to combat fevers.

Most peoples in ancient times respected or worshipped running water, especially springs of pure water. Japanese medical men, the Chinese as well as the Greeks and Romans used baths long before the coming of Christ. Homer suggested the use of warm baths for reducing fatigue, for promoting the healing of wounds and for combating dejection and low spirits.

The Greeks were among the first to appreciate the relationship between physical and mental well-being. They developed centres near springs and rivers using them for bathing and recreation. By 500 BC the transition from mysticism and cult to a logical use of water for physical treatment had occurred. The Romans, with their skills in construction, developed and expanded upon the Greek system of athletics followed by a cold plunge and produced a series of baths ranging from the coldarium through the tepidarium to the frigidarium. The baths were centres where intellectual, recreational activities, health and hygiene were pursued.

Around AD 330 some of these baths were used solely for healing purposes and treatment was indicated first of all for symptoms of rheumatic disease, paralysis and the after effects of injuries. Burns were treated in prolonged baths. There was a decrease in the use of the baths as the Roman Empire declined. The standard of hygiene and morals were lowered. Thus, the early Christians banned the use of the public baths, and the church in the Middle Ages condemned the use of physical forces, such as water, as associated with paganism. The suppression of hydrotherapy in the West was sustained more or less through medieval times but by the 15th, 16th and 17th centuries the use of water for healing purposes acquired some recognition from a few European physicians.

Early pioneers of hydrotherapy were Sir John Floyer who wrote a treatise in 1697 'An enquiry into the right use and abuse of hot, cold and temperate baths'; John Wesley, the founder of Methodism, who published a book on hydrotherapy in 1747 called it 'An easy and natural way of curing most diseases' and Dr Wright who in 1779 published a work on the use of cold in small pox. In the main, however, the academic clinicians at this time were busy diagnosing diseases and working on wards and in the dissecting rooms. Natural therapy hardly concerned them at all. A Silesian peasant, Vincent Pressnitz, had plenty of time and plenty of water. He set up outdoor baths in a woodland setting and placed his clients on treatment programmes that included cold douches, massage and chopping wood. The medical profession viewed his success with concern and tried to put a stop to the craze. During this period a Bavarian priest, Sebastian Kniepp became well known for his water cures. In America, Dr Joel Shaw developed a more systematic water cure at his hydropathic establishment in New York. Professor Winterwitz of Vienna dedicated his life to the scientific study of the practice of hydratics and gave an accurate foundation to modern hydrotherapy.

Advances in the use of water continued in Europe but America lagged behind during the 19th century. However, the warm bath gradually gained popularity and was used in decubiti and other surgical, neuralgic and psychiatric conditions (Kamenetz, 1963). Dr Simon Baruch who worked with Professor Winterwitz furthered the use of hydrotherapy through his work which revolved round the fact that heat or cold was conveyed to the central nervous system by the cutaneous nerves and thus became reflected in the motor pathways. Hydrogymnastics or underwater exercise in warm water was advised in the late 19th century. However, it was not until the first Hubbard tank was made in the 1920s that therapeutic pool exercises really began to be developed systematically.

The two World Wars, especially the second, highlighted the need for the use of water for exercise and the maintenance of fitness and acted as precursors for the current resurgence of the use of the hydrotherapy pool using total immersion as a means of rehabilitation for a wide range of conditions (Harris, 1963).

Today, the ever increasing popularity and value of hydrotherapy appears to be highlighted by an upsurge in research into many different aspects of water, the physiology of exercise in water and so on. Recognition of the ways in which the characteristics and properties of water may be used to create techniques that enhance activity in the water as an integral part of the total physical and psychological care of many and varied conditions will ensure the place of hydrotherapy in their total rehabilitation.

HYDRODYNAMICAL PRINCIPLES

When undertaking hydrotherapy the physiotherapist should have knowledge of the properties and characteristics of water. The physical properties include mass, weight, density, specific gravity, buoyancy, hydrostatic pressure, surface tension, refraction and viscosity (Reid Campion, 1985).

The principles have been described in the literature and the majority of physiotherapists will be familiar with them (Macdonald, 1973; Massey, 1979; Skinner and Thomson, 1983; Davis and Harrison, 1988). It is not the author's intention to describe them further except where the laws of hydrodynamics have especial relevance to the following chapters where specific techniques and exercises are advocated in the text. The hydrodynamic principles which are of particular importance are those related to relative density, turbulence, metacentre, friction and hydrostatic pressure.

Relative Density

Archimedes' principle states that when a body is immersed in a fluid it experiences a buoyant force equal to the weight of the fluid which the body has displaced. The relative density of water is taken as a ratio of one. Any object with a density of less than one will therefore float.

The relative density of the human body varies with age, the young child having a total relative density of approximately 0.86. In adolescence and early adulthood, the relative density of the body increases to approximately 0.97. Later in life the body tends to acquire more adipose tissue (Smith and Bierman, 1973) and the relative density tends to return towards 0.86. It can be seen therefore, that at certain times in the human being's life it is easier to float, and at others harder to float in water.

Each individual part and tissue of the body has its own relative density. The upper limbs are usually less dense than the lower limbs thus the arms float more readily whilst legs tend to sink. The importance of observing and analysing the density of the person undertaking hydrotherapy becomes apparent and should form part of the assessment of that person. Some disabilities, such as paraplegia or Guillain Barré syndrome have marked alterations in density of body parts which have to be taken into account in treatment.

Turbulence

Bernoulli's theorem is concerned with the relation between fluid pressure and fluid velocity along a streamline in the steady flow of a frictionless fluid which has a constant density. Part of the theorem is an expression of energy. The total energy of a particle of water of any moment is the sum of its energies, which are:
- pressure energy
- potential energy
- kinetic energy

Turbulence is the term which denotes the eddies that follow in the wake of an object moving through a fluid. The degree of turbulence will depend on the speed of the movement. If the movement is slow then the flow of the particles is almost parallel to the object and proceeds in smooth continuous curves. Faster movements produce eddies and the energy in these eddies is dissipated, reducing the pressure and increasing the drag on the body. The shape of the body greatly influences the production of turbulence.

Since any movement creates turbulence it may be used in hydrotherapy both to assist and resist movement. The physiotherapist needs to understand the effects of turbulence not only in relation to the patient, but also in relation to her movements around the person being treated in order not to cause a loss of balance. Coping with the effects of turbulence demands balance and coordination and this can be used to develop these skills as part of a treatment programme.

Metacentre

The metacentric principle is concerned with balance in water. A body immersed in water is subjected to two opposing forces—gravity and buoyancy. Gravity acts in a downwards direction, buoyancy in an upwards direction. If these two forces are equal and opposite to one another then the body is balanced and no movement takes place. However, if the forces of gravity and buoyancy are unequal and unaligned, then movement occurs and that movement is always one of rotation. The rotation continues until the two forces are once more in alignment.

When these forces are applied to the human body it can be seen that when floating, the body is balanced and in equilibrium. However, if a part of the body is taken above the surface of the water the balance of the body is upset as the forces of gravity and buoyancy are no longer equal and directionally opposite. The body will rotate until the two forces are aligned once more.

Any movement of the limbs, trunk and head which alters the body shape whether above or below the surface of the water, will produce rotational effects, as will any alteration in shape due to disability. Thus control of the rotations that occur is an important factor during activity in water. The physiotherapist needs to observe and analyse the shape of the person entering water for hydrotherapy and be able to instruct in regard to the appropriate actions to be taken to counteract the rotational effects. It must be understood that these can occur in the vertical as well as the horizontal positions.

Friction

Two scientists Froude (1810–79) and Zahm (1862–1945) directed their work towards the measurement of skin friction of a body passed through water and through air. They found that under similar conditions skin friction was proportional to the densities of the two fluids. Skin friction was found to be 790 times greater in water than air. The amount of energy required to perform a movement in water is in a ratio of 790:1. It can be appreciated that this factor impedes movement and has an important part to play in hydrotherapy. It provides a situation where more active exercise can be undertaken. Along with the impedance to movement as a result of turbulence it also damps down jerky and involuntary movements. If balance is lost, the falling action is retarded and there is time for the person to exert voluntary control to regain the original position.

Hydrostatic Pressure

Pascal's law states that fluid pressure is exerted equally at any level in a horizontal direction, that is, pressure is equal at a constant depth. An immersed body thus has fluid pressure exerted on all surfaces when at rest at a given depth.

However, pressure increases with depth and with the density of the fluid. Since the pressure is equal in all directions at a given depth it is felt evenly on all surfaces of the body. The increased pressure at greater depths may be used to reduce swelling more effectively if the part being treated is in as deep water as possible. This pressure also proves useful in smoothing out jerky movements and increasing coordination if activity is carried out well below the surface. A feeling of weightlessness is brought about through the lateral pressure that is applied combined with the effects of buoyancy.

THE TEMPERATURE OF WATER FOR EXERCISE

Whenever exercise is undertaken certain physiological effects occur. In water these physiological effects of exercise are combined with those brought about by the warmth of the water. In addition, the results of buoyancy and hydrostatic pressure must be considered when the whole body is immersed (Franchimont *et al.*, 1983).

The thermoregulatory system of the body needs to be efficient to cope with exercise in warm water. The hypothalamus responds to the stimulation of the cutaneous thermoreceptors or to the temperature of the blood passing through it. When immersed in water the natural mechanisms for losing heat, such as evaporation, are rendered largely ineffective, since only those parts of the body not under water can lose heat by sweating. As the patient exercises there is increased heating to further compound the problem of losing heat.

The body has elaborate mechanisms for the maintenance of thermal homeostasis. Heat dissipation is balanced against the heat gained from the body's metabolic activities and from the environment. The temperature of the human being is not uniform and varies with the body's ability to transfer heat from the area to which it is applied. Under normal circumstances the heat regulating mechanisms maintain the body temperature within narrow limits. In comfortable surroundings the skin temperature of the head and torso is 33.3°C (92°F) which according to Finnerty and Corbitt (1960) is the point of thermal indifference of the skin for water. On exposure to a hot environment subcutaneous temperatures rise most rapidly in the peripheral parts of the body so that the difference in temperature between the torso and the extremities is obliterated. In warm water, heat loss is limited so a systemic rise in temperature occurs.

Throughout the literature on hydrotherapy there is wide variation as to the temperature at which water should be kept in the hydrotherapy pool. Skinner and Thomson (1983) advocate an average temperature between 35.5°C–36.6°C (96–98°F). Whilst accepting that pool temperatures will vary with the different conditions treated in the hydrotherapy department and according to local environmental factors, Bolton and Goodwin (1974) suggest that the water temperature should be between 34.4°C (94°F) and 37.8°C (100°F).

Davis and Harrison (1988) recommend a range between 35°C and 37°C (95–98.6°F) although as they point out the temperature should be set so that it is suitable for the majority of people using the pool—both patients and physiotherapists. Maintaining the temperature at a required level between 33–37°C (92–98°F) is advised by Golland (1981) although this author also proposes varying temperature ranges for different age groups and conditions. For instance, patients in a younger age bracket with orthopaedic problems could be treated at a lower temperature whilst the older person and those with rheumatic conditions are considered to require a temperature as high as 37°C (98°F).

Huddleston (1961) believed a pool temperature of 30.5–33.3°C (87–92°F) was ideal for therapeutic exercise and general physical programmes providing both sedative and stimulating effects. Palmer (1978, p. 111) argues that 'the thermal effects of hydrotherapy depend on the exact temperature of the pool' and advocates variations in the temperature of the water from summer to winter 32–33°C (89.3–91.2°F) in the former and 34°C (92.6°F) in the latter. This was possibly taking into account the environmental factors pertaining to Queensland, Australia, but nevertheless shows that in cooler ranges it is possible to treat patients satisfactorily.

The work of Finnerty and Corbitt (1960) shows that 33.3°C (92°F) is neutral and has a sedative effect. Temperatures just above this are warm yet still produce sedation, but when the heat rises above 35.5°C (96°F) and upwards the effects are stimulating and temperature is into the hot range. These authors propose that 28.8°C (84°F) is tepid and that below 26.6°C (80°F) produces stimulating effects.

When working with ante- and postnatal women in water exercise programmes Vleminckx (1988) advocates a temperature range between 30–32°C (86–89.6°F). The advantage of this range especially at the highest point is that it allows for relaxation and permits activities to take place at a more leisurely pace. When the water is cooler it is important that exercise is carried out at a faster rate. The information cited above provides sufficient evidence of the variations and requirements of temperature thought necessary by a number of authors. The advocates of higher temperature ranges express concern for the patient and physiotherapist alike and propose shorter treatment sessions in the water, packing following treatment and other measures.

The work of Franchimont *et al.* (1983) stresses that temperatures above 35°C (95°C) are disadvantageous as the beneficial effects of treatment in warm water are dissipated due to alterations in the cardio-vascular system which may produce untoward consequences. Higher temperatures do produce relaxation but when patients are subjected to more than 15–20 min in water heated to 35°C (95°F) or above they become ennervated, tired and frequently sleep for up to three hours following treatment. Koga (1985) found that a neutral water temperature for light exercise was 31°C (87.4°F) and that light exercise in temperatures of 27°C (80.3°F), 31°C (87.4°F) and 35°C (95°F) showed no discrepancies as far as the thermal response of the body was concerned.

All the desired effects of hydrotherapy for the neurological patient, such as relaxation of muscles, decrease of pain which is a result of muscle spasm, the improvement in the circulation and the removal of waste metabolic products from hypertonic muscle groups are considered by Palmer (1978) to be achieved in water temperatures ranging from 32°C (89.3°F) to 34°C (92.6°F). Furthermore, Palmer suggests that to work with neurological conditions in water where the temperature is above 34°C (92.6°F) will produce debilitating consequences for the patient as well as the physiotherapist.

Tenseness may be brought about in the neurological patient by work in water that is too cool, that is, below 32°C (89.3°F) (Palmer, 1978). According to Vleminckx (1988) when water is too cold the response of the skin thermoreceptors is reduced and an increase in tone may occur due to stimulation of the motor neurons. There are those physiotherapists who would argue that the geographical location may have an influence in deciding at what temperature the water should be kept. Since most hydrotherapy pools are enclosed this argument would appear to have little weight. Where an outdoor pool is used it may well be that a variation in temperature between summer and winter would be considered. In tropical and sub-tropical climates the pool temperature might range between 34–35°C (92.6–98.6°F) in winter to 31–33°C (87.4–92°F) in summer.

It is impractical to change the temperature of the water, and in hydrotherapy pools where a variety of conditions and age groups are treated it is impossible to vary it to suit everyone. Golland

(1981) recommends a water temperature range between 35–36°C (95–97°F) to cover all contingencies.

However, in this author's experience the pool water should be heated to a range between 32°C (89.6°F) and 34°C (93.2°F). This caters for all conditions, avoids any debilitating or untoward effects provided that all contra-indications to hydrotherapy have been considered. In the past, and in many pools even today, the trend of keeping the water temperature in the higher ranges goes against research findings, ignores the thermal indifference of the skin temperature and puts patients and physiotherapists at risk.

PHYSIOTHERAPIST AND THE HYDROTHERAPY POOL

Considerations which must be taken into account when undertaking hydrotherapy treatment are the type of exercise and the severity, in addition to the duration of the programme on any one day. These must be studied in relation to the water temperature. If this is high then exercises need to be modified and the session shortened if the patient is to avoid untoward effects and post treatment care needs to be carefully monitored.

Patients can only be satisfactorily treated by the physiotherapist who is in the water. This is confirmed by Davis and Harrison (1988). Certainly techniques such as the Bad Ragaz patterns can only be carried out by the patient and physiotherapist working together in the pool. Other techniques require attention to detail, the correct attachment of floats, monitoring of muscle work, specialized techniques and the general care and handling of the patient. In any case it seems wrong to expect patients—especially those in the older age group who may not swim, or may have an anxiety about water—to go into the pool where buoyancy and rotational effects occur that can so easily upset the balance thus producing untoward responses and actions whilst the physiotherapist stays on the poolside.

For the physiotherapist, high temperatures reduce the ability to carry out effective treatments and decrease the time that can be spent in the water. Generally speaking two to three hours in the pool in any one day is sufficient, particularly if the physiotherapist is working in the hydrotherapy department for several weeks or months at a time. It is advisable to divide the time spent in the water into sessions. If working three hours a day, then two 1½ hour sessions with reasonable breaks between each is acceptable. Skinner and Thomson (1983) suggest 20–30 minutes is adequate time to recover $1\frac{1}{2}$ hours in the water. A longer period for recovery is preferable. Davis and Harrison (1988) believe that 2 hours in the water is possible and should not be exceeded if the physiotherapist is working an extended tour of duty in the pool.

In this author's experience especially when the warmth of the water is in the higher ranges it is advantageous for the physiotherapist to emerge from the pool to bring in each patient. Not only is there time for some cooling to take place, but it provides an opportunity to observe the patient and to note asymmetry of shape. Analysis of the rotational effects likely to occur means that the patient can be informed about these and instructed in the actions to take to counteract the rotations as he enters the water. Thus the patient becomes more adjusted to water activity. Such mental adjustment is extended as the programme progresses (see page 17).

It is not possible to have these short times out of the water when conducting classes and in these instances physiotherapists need to gradually adjust by initially taking shorter sessions. Individually, physiotherapists vary in their reaction to the water, and to temperature, but no one person should undertake longer periods in the water than those advocated earlier. When the water temperature is high, that is, above 35°C (95°F) and if the physiotherapist spends two or more hours twice a day in the water there is a build up of fatigue and tiredness that at the end of two weeks may result in extreme reactions such as sleeping for as long as 24 hours. Whilst the majority of authors agree that the temperature of the pool area should be lower than that of the water and the changing and rest rooms should be below that of the pool area each presents a different range.

Bolton and Goodwin (1974) advocate 21°C (70°F) for change areas; Skinner and Thomson (1983) suggest 25°C (78°F) for the pool area and four degrees below that for the other areas, whilst Davis and Harrison (1988) recommend a temperature as low as 18.5°C (65°F) for the rest areas. Proper temperature control and good ventilation are essential if the ideal temperature and a humidity of between 50–60% is to be maintained.

ASSESSMENT AND RECORDING

It is common practice to assess patients for physiotherapy treatment programmes on land and to record details of the treatment session in the patient's records. However, such practices are less regular when hydrotherapy treatments are undertaken. Frequently, the land assessment is considered adequate information on which to base the water programme (Harrison, 1980). In such instances no account is taken of the nature of the medium or of the special effects that result from the fact that on entering the water the body is acted upon by two forces simultaneously—namely, gravity or downthrust and buoyancy or upthrust.

As Davis and Harrison (1988) so rightly stress translating dry land procedures to water denies the uniqueness of the medium and fails to capitalize on this factor for the benefit of the patient. An assessment carried out on land cannot take into account the effects of buoyancy on a movement. For instance, a patient with a problem involving the shoulder joint may only be able to abduct the arm from the side to 40° on land, but in the pool with buoyancy assisting the movement may obtain a greater range. This additional range may be achieved on land as an assisted active movement or with the limb in suspension, but is still not applicable as a baseline for the hydrotherapy programme.

All programmes, hydrotherapy programmes included, should have realistic aims, but such aims must be related to the medium in which activity is to take place.

A land assessment is essential and the details should be noted by the physiotherapist taking the patient for treatment in the water. An assessment based on the same format should be carried out for water, but a number of additional points with particular relevance to activity in water being taken into consideration.

Assessment

This assessment procedure follows the system in use at the School of Physiotherapy, Curtin University of Technology in Western Australia.

The format is based on the SOAP assessment (Weed, 1971), but has been expanded to SOAPIER (Hastings L., 1983 Personal Communication). It is used for land and water assessments.

Method of Recording Physiotherapy Assessment and Treatment

The initials SOAPIER are derived from the following;

S: Subjective assessment—information given by the patients about themselves.

O: Objective assessment—examination of the patient.

A: Analysis of the above information—diagnosis and medical history and S and O to formulate a problem list.

P: Plan of action—for each of the problems.

I: Intervention—treatment of the patient.

E: Evaluation—evaluation of the intervention; what occurred as the result of treatment.

R: Review—the next treatment session and any proposed treatment changes.

These details are suitable for both land and water, but certain factors must be elicited that relate specifically to water.

S: Subjective assessment—must include the patient's attitude to water, information as to their perceived ability in water, and details of previous hydrotherapy or other water activity such as type, place, date and results.

O: Objective assessment—takes into account the shape and density of the patient as well as any contradictions to hydrotherapy.

A: Analysis—the analysis of shape and density is vital and forms part of the problem list.

I: Intervention—will also include the teaching of mental adjustment, balance restoration and rotational control.

E: Evaluation.

R: Review.

For ongoing management the SOAPIER format is used as appropriate and is divided into two parts.

1. The acute/short-term patient.
2. The chronic/long-term patient.

For the acute/short-term patient a daily SOIER is conducted and a new A and P formulated as the S and O alter. For the chronic/long-term patient IER is carried out and a full SOAPIER takes place weekly. Any assessment for water should take in the suitability of a patient for group activity as it may be necessary to involve people in group hydrotherapy sessions (p. 31). Without adequate assessment hydrotherapy programmes tailored to the individual's needs are not possible. Continuous assessment ensures progression and improved and faster recovery of the condition.

The progression of exercise in water is markedly different from that on land and fine progressions of techniques are possible (Skinner and Thomson, 1983). This applies not only to buoyancy assisted, buoyancy neutral and buoyancy resisted exercises, but to other procedures such as Bad Ragaz patterns, hold-relax, repeated contractions and exercises based on the combined effects of buoyancy, turbulence and metacentric principles, or each of these used separately.

Recording

Detailed recording of hydrotherapy treatments is as important as documentation of other treatments. The following items should be included:

- the length of the treatment
- the temperature of the water
- the depths used
- the exercises, patterns included in the programme
- any progressions of the exercises
- any improvements in the patient's condition and activity
- any untoward effects
- individual and/or group treatment.

Some hospital departments and centres may have other items they specifically need included in their records of treatment.

There is no doubt that only by accurate and comprehensive assessment and recording will it be possible to prove the effectiveness of hydrotherapy. Currently, there is a dearth of evaluative material, most of the comments about the value of hydrotherapy treatments are subjective. If careful and conscientious assessment and recording is carried out they will not only enhance the programmes themselves, but enable physiotherapists to promote hydrotherapy and ensure it takes its place in the overall rehabilitation of the many conditions treated in water.

ANALYSIS OF SHAPE AND DENSITY, MENTAL ADJUSTMENT AND BALANCE RESTORATION

The importance of observing and analysing body shape and density, should not be under-estimated. It has a bearing on the mental adjustment of the person undertaking activity in water, their security in the medium, on their willingness to cooperate with the physiotherapist in carrying out the required activities and on the exercise programme itself. Time spent in helping the person acquire the skills of vertical and lateral rotational control is never wasted and leads to happy and productive treatment sessions.

Discussion of the objective aspect of the SOAPIER format for assessment indicates the need for the observation of the patient's shape and density. The factors of shape and density are critical in response to immersion in water. Water reacts to the shape and density of any object placed in it and floats the object according to these factors. When applied to a human being the variations in shape and density of different parts of the body account for the many and varied balance positions. Each body part has its own relative density. The sum of these usually adds up to a density less than the weight of water thus the human body mostly floats. However, some body parts are less dense than others; these will tend to float more easily, whilst the denser parts will tend to sink.

All human beings are asymmetrical to a greater or lesser degree and will have a balance problem in water. In the person with a medical condition or disability the alteration in shape and/or density will be more marked. The importance of observing shape and density and analysing the effects when in the water cannot be stressed too strongly. The physiotherapist should observe the person anteriorly, posteriorly, laterally and longitudinally. With knowledge of the likely rotation effects that will occur to the analysed shape the physiotherapist can commence mentally adjusting the person prior to entering the water by instructing them in the action to take to control the movement of rotation.

Mental Adjustment

Once in the water and at an appropriate depth upon which the person's condition has some bearing further mental adjustment can take place. The ability to blow the water away from the mouth adds to security of mind. Facing each other the physiotherapist demonstrates the blowing action. With their hands on the physiotherapist's shoulders for support the person demonstrates a similar action repeating it several times until it has become a more automatic response.

An understanding that water has weight and can be leant on and used as a force against which work can take place, helps in furthering mental adjustment. To develop this knowledge the physiotherapist adopts a similar position facing the person whose hands are on the physiotherapist's shoulders. The physiotherapist's hands are on either side of the person's waist with the fingers pointing away. The first action is to lean to one side with the shoulders and head and then to lean to the other side. The shoulders must be beneath the surface of the water. Once the feeling of being able to push against the water has been established it can be further stressed by taking several steps, if possible in a sitting position, first to one side and then the other, the head and shoulders leading the movement.

Balance Restoration

The ability to restore the body's balance should be developed around the two rotations that occur in water—vertical and lateral.

Vertical rotation—occurs in a forward and backward direction around the body's centre of buoyancy and incorporates the ability to recover to the upright position from either supine or prone lying. It is a skill that is required for total independence in the water and demonstrates the ability to recover to a safe breathing position.

To achieve supine lying, the head is taken slowly backwards and the feet will slowly rise to the surface, the feet moving forward and upwards. Recovery from this position requires strong flexion of the cervical spine, trunk, hips and knees, with flexion of the shoulders in abduction followed by precise balance of the head over the body to maintain the upright position.

To achieve prone lying, the head is taken slowly forwards, while the legs move backward and upward to the surface. Recovery from this position to the upright may be achieved by laterally rotating onto the back and then affecting a forward recovery. Alternatively, the head may be strongly extended, the hips and knees flexed, and when the body is vertical the legs then extended and the body balanced precisely by the head in the upright position.

Apart from the feeling of security, the ability to perform vertical rotation proves useful when placing patients on a submerged plinth, or in flotation equipment. It has also implications for developing balance and coordination in a variety of conditions, such as the head injured and the paraplegic patient. Additionally, the ability to create vertical rotation can be used in a number of specific exercises.

Lateral rotation—takes place in two planes. The rotational movement occurs around the longitudinal axis of the body. In the vertical position by using the head and arms the human being is able to create a lateral or turning movement in the upright position. When lying in the water the head, arms and legs, either singly or collectively, can be used to create a lateral or turning rotation around the longitudinal axis of the body.

Instruction in the techniques of creating or controlling lateral rotation in both positions aids the mental adjustment of the person giving a sense of security and confidence. If such instruction follows on the acquisition of vertical rotation described above lateral rotation and vertical may be combined so that the person can always return to a safe breathing position. Should the person fall forward in the water it is possible to rotate on to the back and then perform vertical rotation to achieve the upright position once more. When teaching the skill of lateral or turning movement it is essential that rolling is taught in both directions that is, to the right and left sides. It can also be developed in an extended as well as flexed pattern.

In extension the movements of the horizontal body are to turn the head to the side to which the roll is being directed whilst the arm and leg on the opposite side are brought across the body. If rotating in a flexed posture the head and arms repeat the action for the extended posture whilst both the legs may be flexed and rotated towards the side to which the head is turned. The amount of flexion in the legs can vary from leg to leg depending on the condition being treated. For example, whilst treating a patient with a low back pain problem recently it was found advantageous to teach rolling as this action presented considerable difficulty in bed. With considerable lack of mobility in the whole back and a marked tendency to hold the spine extended it was found that encouraging this rotation from one arm of the physiotherapist to the other arm (Reid Campion, 1985) in a flexed posture, broke the extended pattern demonstrated by the patient and developed some gentle rotation between the shoulder and pelvic girdles without any detrimental effects.

With the acquisition of the skills of vertical and lateral rotation the person is well adjusted to water and consequently exercises in a more effective manner. If possible a floating position should be developed. This can be achieved by altering the shape of the person through changing the position of the legs and arms and thus altering the centre of gravity and buoyancy. An extension of this would be to encourage independent bilateral movement through the water. A sculling action is recommended for the arms and a modified back stroke kick for the legs.

Armed with a knowledge and understanding of water and the actions to take if the body's balance is disturbed for any reason, the patient is reassured and has a greater pleasure in the use of water in the rehabilitation programme.

REFERENCES

Bolton E., Goodwin D. (1974). *An Introduction to Pool Exercises*, Edinburgh: Churchill Livingstone.

Davis, B.C., Harrison, R.A. (1988). *Hydrotherapy in Practice*, Edinburgh: Churchill Livingstone.

Franchimont P., Juchmes J., Lecomte J. (1983). Hydrotherapy Mechanisms and Indications. *Pharmac. Ther.*, **20**, 79–93.

Finnerty F.G., Corbitt T. (1960). *Hydrotherapy*, London: Ungar.

Golland A. (1981). Basic hydrotherapy, *Physiotherapy*, **67**, (9); 258–262.

Harris R. (1963). Therapeutic pools In *Medical Hydrology* (Licht S. ed.) New Haven: Elizabeth Licht Publisher.

Harrison R.A. (1980). Hydrotherapy in rheumatic conditions. In *Physiotherapy in Rheumatology* (Hyde S.A. ed.), Oxford: Blackwell Scientific Publications.

Huddleston O.L. (1961). *Hydrotherapy in Therapeutic Exercises*, Philadelphia: F.A. Davis.

Kamenetz H.L. (1963). History of American spas and hydrotherapy. In *Medical Hydrology*, (Licht S. ed.). New Haven: Elisabeth Licht Publisher.

Koga, S. (1985). The regional difference of thermal response to immersion during rest and exercise. *Annals Physiol. Anthrop.*, **4**(2), 191–192.

Krizek V. (1963). History of balenotherapy. In *Medical Hydrology*, (Licht S. ed.). New Haven: Elizabeth Licht Publisher.

MacDonald F. (1973). *Mechanics for Movement*, London: G. Bell and Sons.

Massey B.S. (1979). *Mechanics of Fluids*, 4th edn., New York: Van Nostrand Reinhold Company.

Palmer R.P. (1978). *Guidelines to Neurological Rehabilitation*, 2nd edn. Queensland: Multiple Sclerosis Society.

Price R. (1981). Hydrotherapy in England 1840–70, *Medical History*, **25**, 269–280.

Reid Campion M. (1985). *Hydrotherapy in Paediatrics*, Oxford: Heinemann Medical Books.

Skinner A.T., Thomson A.M. eds. (1983). *Duffield's Exercises in Water* 3rd edn. London: Baillière Tindall.

Smith D.W., Bierman E.L. (1973). *The Biological Ages of Man – from conception through to Old Age*, Philadelphia: W.B. Saunders.

Vleminckx M. (1988). Pregnancy and recovery: the aquatic approach in obstetrics and gynaecology. In *Obstetrics and Gynaecology*, (McKenna J. ed.). Edinburgh: Churchill Livingstone.

Weed L.L. (1971). *Medical Records, Medical Education and Patient Care*, Chicago: Year Book Medical Publishers.

Wyman J. (1944). Hydrotherapy in Medical Physics, **1**, pp. 619–622. (Glazer O. ed.). Chicago: Year Book Publishers.

Techniques of Exercise in Water and Therapeutic Swimming

Hydrogymnastics as a systematic form of exercise in water began in the early part of the 20th century (Kamenetz, 1963). The first Hubbard tank, made in 1928, was designed primarily for underwater exercise. Some years earlier, in 1911, Lowman was using such exercise for patients with spasticity, whilst others suffering from anterior poliomyelitis, including Franklin D. Roosevelt, were finding hydrogymnastics in warm water beneficial.

Harris (1963) stresses that hydrotherapy in water should only be conducted by physiotherapists who have been given practical instruction in the techniques of exercise in water. Bennett (1951, p. 513) proposes that 'unless exercise in water is carried out by trained personnel the advantages—motivation, pleasure, novelty and enhancement of movement—may become disadvantages and lead to poor patterns of movement and fatigue.'

It is vital that the physiotherapist appreciates the difference between exercises carried out on land and in water. It is totally inappropriate to use land based exercise in water since the unique properties offered by the medium are neglected and water not used as a modality for rehabilitation in its own right. Exercises in water differ from similar exercises carried out on land. The difference lies in the dissimilarity of the physical properties of the two fluids.

The uniqueness of water lies mainly in the presence of buoyancy. Buoyancy supports the body and diminishes the effects of gravity. An advantage accruing from this is that it induces relaxation and relieves pain, thus the movements a person can perform on land only with difficulty and considerable pain may be used in the hydrotherapy programme where pain is eased and where the weightlessness allows a greater freedom of movement. Other factors are cohesion, viscosity, turbulence and friction. Describing cohesion and viscosity Harris and McInnes (1963) state that these factors provide resistance to all movements in the water. Other authors use the term resistance (Bolton and Goodwin, 1974; Skinner and Thomson, 1983) whilst Davis and Harrison (1988) write of resistance but also refer to the bow wave effect impeding movement. For some years the author of this chapter has advocated the use of the word impedance as more suitable than resistance.

Resistance implies the solidity of an object such as the resistances against which the human being works on land. For example, for a person to achieve the standing position from sitting the floor is used against which to thrust. Such resistance is not present in water, especially when in deeper water or in the horizontal position where there is no 'resistance' to thrust against, but movement is impeded by cohesion, viscosity, turbulence and frictional forces. The degree to which movement through water is impeded also depends on the speed of the action and the shape of the object.

In the editor's and authors' opinions the physiotherapist should be in the water when treating patients (see p. 12). For a number of reasons it is undesirable to expect patients to go into the water whilst the physiotherapist remains on land. Most techniques require that the physiotherapist is in the water with the patient; the exercises that can be taught from the bathside are usually carried out less effectively if the physiotherapist instructs from dry land. Risk factors are compounded when the physiotherapist is not in the pool. The advantages of the physiotherapist's presence in the water far outweight the disadvantages.

THERAPEUTIC EFFECTS OF EXERCISE IN WATER

The therapeutic effects of exercise in water have been well documented (Skinner and Thomas, 1983; Davis and Harrison, 1988). It is recognized that an increase in muscle power and endurance, the mobilizing of joints, the reduction of spasticity, relaxation, improvements in balance and coordination, functional activity and recreation are amongst the most important of these effects.

Techniques of Exercise in Water

There are a number of techniques of exercise in water available to the physiotherapist. These include:
- buoyancy assisted, supported, resisted, exercise
- Bad Ragaz patterns
- hold–relax techniques
- stabilizations

- repeated contractions
- breathing exercises

and techniques based on hydrodynamical principles. In some instances the laws governing buoyancy and balance in water are involved; in others the three principles—buoyancy, turbulence and balance—are incorporated. These techniques either produce movement as a reaction, enhance movement and/or develop balance and coordination.

Buoyancy assisted, supported, resisted exercise

These are the most commonly used exercises carried out in the hydrotherapy pool. They are usually carried out with the patient lying supported on a submerged plinth or in flotation equipment or in the sitting and standing position, when the patient may hold the rail for support and stability.

The starting position for each exercise is important as on this will depend whether the movement has buoyancy either assisting, supporting, or resisting it. In these exercises the physiotherapist endeavours to isolate the movement and this may be achieved by providing suitable floats above the joint being exercised or by the physiotherapist giving manual assistance. With the hands involved in this way the physiotherapist cannot give manual assistance or resistance to the patient's movement which is frequently required.

The four main starting positions of standing, sitting, kneeling and lying can be varied enormously (Bolton and Goodwin, 1974; Skinner and Thomson, 1983). There is little advantage to be gained from reiterating the variations here, but it is important to stress that depending on the effects of buoyancy required these must be understood if this type of exercise is to be effectively executed and the progression of exercise obtained. Apart from the starting position the commands to the patient are important so that the correct movement takes place. It is all too easy to involve other body parts due to the difficulty of acquiring stability in water so attention to detail is essential. Progression of this type of exercise can be further obtained by altering the lever arm, adding floats, the speed and range of movement as well as the number of repetitions.

Bad Ragaz patterns

Bad Ragaz patterns were originally developed in Germany, but have been adapted and developed at Bad Ragaz in Switzerland.

This technique utilizes the properties of water, for instance, buoyancy is needed for flotation only, whilst the bow wave and drag effects provide the impedance to movement. The patterns themselves allow normal anatomical and physiological movements involving the joints and muscles concerned in the movements.

The bow wave effect demonstrates an increase in pressure ahead of the direction of movement whilst the drag effect occurs behind the direction of movement. By varying both the bow wave and drag effect, impedance to movement can be varied.

Bad Ragaz patterns can only be carried out if the physiotherapist is in the water handling and instructing the patient. There are three ways in which the physiotherapist acts in relation to the patient. They are

- the physiotherapist providing fixation whilst the patient moves through the water—either towards, away from or around the physiotherapist
- the physiotherapist acts as the stabilizing factor but this moves and the patient is pushed in the direction of movement which leads to an increase in impedance to the movement
- the patient holds a fixed position whilst being pushed through the water by the physiotherapist.

These points highlight the need for the stability and flexibility of the physiotherapist. To ensure these factors are developed the physiotherapist should not work in a depth greater than that of the level of the 8th thoracic vertebra.

Holds should be precise and capable of guiding the patient to work the required muscle groups of the mass pattern of a limb or trunk. Holds can also provide resistance to movement so that stronger components can be developed—irradiation or overflow carried over to the weaker muscle groups. It is possible to vary the hold from proximal to distal positions on the limbs. Proximal holds give the physiotherapist greater control and there is increased security for the patient, and such a hold would be employed when the pattern involves movement of a possible painful joint. Distal holds allow greater ranges of movement and encourage increased muscle work.

The starting positions for Bad Ragaz patterns are supine lying, side lying or prone lying. Patterns provide both isotonic and isometric muscle work and have been devised for the upper and lower limbs and trunk. The Bad Ragaz patterns allow the physiotherapist and patient to work together in enjoyable cooperation and the strength of the movement can be carefully monitored and graded.

As the individual patterns have been well documented (Skinner and Thomson, 1983; Davis and Harrison, 1988) it is not proposed to detail them here. The usual patterns can be adapted and modified and as the physiotherapist becomes skilled in their use she will find it possible to devise and develop her own variations.

Hold–relax techniques

Hold–relax techniques in water are similar to those carried out on land except that the patient must be positioned so that buoyancy assists movement into the required range.

Stabilization

The freedom of movement which is possible in water is the only difference between this technique on land and in water. It is used to produce co-contraction of a joint which has implications for balance and coordination in addition to increasing muscle strength and improving the circulation to painful joints.

Repeated contractions

This technique involves isometric and isotonic work and when used in water movement and the 'holding' component can be developed against turbulent effect or a combination of turbulence and buoyancy. The activity which is repeated permits the weaker components of movement patterns to develop thus increasing the development of strength and stamina.

Breathing exercises

The freedom of movement available in water is used in this technique to develop lateral and posterior costal expansion. The technique involves careful monitoring of the patient's breathing and judiciously applied light stretch. Like all the other specialized techniques listed breathing exercises have been described in detail and the reader is referred to those authors (Skinner and Thomson, 1983; Davis and Harrison, 1988).

Techniques using Buoyancy, Turbulence and Balance in Water

These techniques are based on the hydrodynamical principles of buoyancy, turbulence and balance in water. The techniques may use any or all three of the principles at any one time. For ease of description they are referred to as hydrodynamic exercise in the text, and can only take place in water where the forces of gravity and buoyancy are present and act simultaneously on the body. In any situation balance, coordination, movement, movement control, body image, spatial awareness and reaction to positions, shape, buoyancy and turbulence may be involved.

As already seen water reacts to the shape and density of any object placed in it and floats the object accordingly (Reid Campion, 1985). The variations in the shape and density of human beings account for the myriad of balance positions.

General Principles

The general principles involved in these patterns are that from a position of stability a movement is made, then balance occurs against the turbulent effects created by the movement and further adjustments are made to balance the body in the new posture. Where movements are small and little or no turbulence is created buoyancy and balance are the two principles involved. Where the body is supported by the physiotherapist buoyancy plays a part involved as it is with the balance of the body in water as opposed to gravity, the alteration in shape, particularly if a part of the body is taken above the surface of the water producing a quick and massive rotational response. Controlling this response produces strong muscle work even when the alteration of the shape is small.

Turbulence is felt as a force along the surface of a limb behind the direction of movement, but mainly distally. Small slow movements will create little turbulence, but larger and more rapid movements will create greater turbulence with increased appreciation of the drag effect which impedes movement. This enhances awareness of body image and with the necessity of controlling the body against the disturbing factor of turbulence develops balance and coordination.

Marked alterations in shape and density which occur in disease and disability demand more control to counteract the rotational movement. Such control may be developed in the rehabilitation programme, but should be taught from the beginning. The importance of analysing shape and density has already been discussed. Reference to it has been made at this point to expand on its use as a means of teaching balance and coordination, as well as developing exercises and patterns of movement and control which require precise muscle work. The patterns can be conducted in the four main starting positions—standing, sitting, kneeling and lying. The depth at which they are conducted in the first three of the above starting positions must be appropriate for the patient's condition, ensuring that the water level is not below the xiphisternum where approximately 30% of weight bearing occurs and preferably with the body positioned so that the shoulders are covered by the water so that approximately only 10% of the body weight is borne.

Examples

The following examples will serve to illustrate ways in which these techniques may be developed.

Changing body shapes

Changing body shapes means that water will balance the body in a new position. For instance if the body is collapsed into its smallest shape that of being curled up like a 'ball' (Reid Campion, 1985) water will rotate this shape forward and balance the body over its centre of buoyancy with the thoracic spine visible above the surface of the water.

If the physiotherapist holds the person's curled up body by placing one arm behind and around the waist and placing the other hand over the person's hands which are clasped around the knees it is possible to control the forward movement created by the water (Reid Campion, 1985). The person's curled up body should be held as low as possible in the water so that the shoulders are covered and where the neck is to be treated this should be immersed as deep as is practical. Gentle rocking of the body by the physiotherapist will promote flexion and extension of the cervical spine. It is essential that the water is blown away from the mouth as the head goes forward; this tends to increase the movement of flexion. Such breathing control has been described under mental adjustment and balance restoration.

Tilting the body

By tilting the curled body sideways side flexion of the neck can be obtained.

In neurological conditions where extensor tone is increased in the lower limb(s) and flexor tone increased in the upper limb(s) the curled up or 'ball' position (Reid Campion, 1985) will have the effect of reducing the extensor spasticity in the leg(s) and encourage protraction of the shoulder, extension of the elbow, the mid-position of the forearm and some extension of the wrist and fingers. If the physiotherapist, holding the curled up body as described above, then rocks the person forwards and backwards slowly and rhythmically reduction of increased muscle tone is aided. When the person is required to come out of the curled up posture this should be performed slowly and with the physiotherapist's support. If the erect position is required then the procedure of uncurling should take place in deep water so that as the person attains the erect position the minimum amount of gravity is placed on the patient. Should spasticity return or be a problem it is advisable to let the uncurling take place slowly into supine lying still supported by the physiotherapist.

Rotating the body

Rotation of the cervical spine can be developed if the body is extended into its longest shape; that is, lying with the hands by the sides of the body and supported by the physiotherapist using the horizontal backing hold (Reid Campion, 1985). The body is rolled first in one direction and then the other and the person instructed to bring the body to a flat position again by rotating the head to the opposite side to which the body is being rolled.

Use of turbulence

When retraining gait greater balance and coordination can be developed over and above that achieved with turbulence judi-ciously placed behind the patient to increase the difficulty of forward movement. This can be accomplished by instructing the person to pause and stabilize the body, not letting it be disturbed by turbulent effect created by the movement. If walking is performed in this way, the starting position is standing on one leg with the arms stretched forwards just below the surface of the water, with one leg raised in flexion at the hip, the knee extended and the foot dorsiflexed. The supporting knee should be extended. A step is taken onto the forward leg and the original supporting limb is allowed to extend at the hip, the pelvis facing forwards, so that rotation of the pelvis and trunk does not take place. The steps taken may be small at first, but can be gradually increased. If maintaining balance is difficult in the pauses between each movement, the arms may be moved slowly sideways in abduction from the forward position, thus bringing the centre of gravity back within the body. Once a stable position is achieved, the arms are moved forward in a controlled manner and the next part of the pattern commenced. The extended leg is brought forward with a straight knee and is raised forwards as high as possible. Buoyancy assists the flexion at the hip. The body is stabilized again before the next step is taken.

This 'goose-step' demands considerable control throughout the body, particularly as the size of the stride increases, producing great turbulence. These movements can be extended till eventually the person may jump onto one leg, pause to stabilize the body, before continuing the pattern.

This method of gait retraining has, in the author's experience, proved valuable in many conditions, notably in the orthopaedic and neurological ones. The pattern is not easily learned, and careful instruction is necessary, but the majority of persons treated enjoy both the mental and physical exercise required in the acquisition of the skill. In one instance this gait retraining combined with other techniques developed on similar lines were of particular value in the rehabilitation of a ballet dancer who had suffered severe damage to one knee requiring surgery and prolonged rehabilitation. Progress was excellent and she finally returned to dancing on points with the ballet company.

The 'goose-step' can be varied to stepping and turning so that all the movements of the hips are involved in the pattern combined with trunk, shoulder girdle and head rotation.

Static muscle work

Static muscle work is developed in techniques that utilize a fixed position followed by changes of shape using the lower or upper limbs or both. It is usual to convert one shape to another by repositioning one lower limb and using the arms in varying patterns pausing after each movement to allow the body to be balanced.

Controlling the body shape after each movement produces muscle work that is fine yet strong.

To develop muscle work for the dorsiflexors and plantarflexors of the foot the person may be in the 'sitting' or 'cube' position (Reid Campion, 1985) with the arms forward and the feet about hip width apart, a right angle at the hip, knee and ankle joints. Stretching the fingers forwards will cause the body to rotate forwards and the heels will rise. When sufficient elevation of the heels has occurred extension of the head will bring the body back to the original starting position. To produce dorsiflexion the hips should be allowed to drop towards the heels; this action brings about rotation of the body in a backwards direction. Once sufficient dorsiflexion has been created a forward action of the head will bring the body to the upright 'sitting' position again. Slow rocking forwards and backwards in this position using the actions described, or the extended wrists and hands, just above the surface in a pulling or pushing type action will produce strong muscle work for the dorsiflexors and plantarflexors of the ankle. If only one muscle group is to be exercised then the action which produces the movement is done repeatedly, the person coming back to the original starting position between each movement.

Where knee extension with dorsiflexion requires re-education and training and as a strengthening activity for the quadriceps muscle the 'sitting' position may be utilized again. Extending first one knee and then the other towards the surface, but outside the forward held arms, at the same time dorsiflexing the foot and creating a 'bubble' on the surface. The foot should never break through the surface of the water. The body weight has to be transferred to the supporting side just prior to the kicking action. The person remains in the 'sitting' position with the arms forward all the time. The movements once learnt, can be gradually speeded up so that the shifting of the body weight and the kicking action proceed continuously. As a useful lead into the backstroke kick the kicking action may be brought closer to the arms and so into midline the person gradually lying back as they do so.

The combined use of buoyancy, turbulence and balance in water adds a new dimension to activity in water. These patterns are unique to hydrotherapy as only in water is the body acted upon by two forces simultaneously—the forces of gravity or downthrust and buoyancy or upthrust. A wide range of patterns can be developed. They require that the patient and physiotherapist work closely together particularly where pain is present. In some instances the patient has to be supported by the physiotherapist. In others the physiotherapist must correct the patient's posture and this requires minute attention to the muscle work which changes with each alteration of shape. Reactions, balance, coordination and the enhancement of movement are developed strongly in these patterns.

It can be seen then that the physiotherapist being in the water with the person will produce the best results. Bad Ragaz patterns, successive induction, slow reversals and stabilizations, together with hydrodynamic exercise where the physiotherapist must observe the muscle action and correct any untoward alterations in shape, demand the presence of the physiotherapist in the water. This is also true where turbulent assisted and resisted activity is taking place. The physiotherapist is required to create turbulence in appropriate areas in relation to the person's body. Much is made of the time factor but in the author's experience the advantages of effective treatment far outweigh any disadvantages. A session for a number of persons being treated at the same time can be appropriately timetabled to include both group and individual work (p 32). It is sad to reflect that in some instances people are given a few instructions about exercise in water for their condition and are then left to carry them out with little or no supervision nor any attempt to evaluate and progress the programme.

GROUP WORK

Working in groups has been shown to have considerable advantages. Motivation, socialization and the ability to work longer with great concentration are amongst these advantages (Cotton and Kinsman, 1983) and these are brought about by classwork in the water just as in group work on land.

- the patient gains confidence from working with others
- a feeling of fellowship develops
- patients take some responsibility for their own treatment
- patients become more extrovert
- concentrate less on their own problems and tend to set standards for each other.

The suitability of a patient to participate in classwork should form part of the original assessment and later evaluation. Classwork may not be appropriate initially for some patients, but as they progress it may be possible for them to be included. Some of the techniques of exercise, for example, the Bad Ragaz patterns are not suitable for group work due to a lack of the one-to-one relationship required and to the space factor. Where staffing is a problem group work often means more patients can be treated by one or two physiotherapists.

There is a place for both individual and group treatment and many patients can benefit from both during each session of water activity. In the author's experience it is useful to gather the patients together as they enter the pool and conduct some general exercises all together at the beginning of the session. If these exercises are conducted to music the activity becomes more pleasurable. Individual treatment can be carried out following the early group work and gathering together again towards the end of the session as a 'wind down' is valuable. On the whole patients should be able to manage on their own in the water; this is important where there is only one physiotherapist to a group. However, judicious positioning of the more able patients in relation to those who are less able frequently eases the situation. The disadvantages of too large a group are familiar and regulating the number of participants in a group must be uppermost in the physiotherapist's mind. Too large a group can disadvantage all. Precise and accurate movement should not be sacrificed in classes; if there is a large number of participants it is difficult to monitor everybody's actions.

Group work is suitable for most conditions, but probably more so for orthopaedic and rheumatic conditions. Patients with neurological problems can also enjoy participation in group work although the more severely disabled, such as the head-injured, require a one-to-one basis with a physiotherapist within the group situation. In the ensuing chapters group work for different conditions is discussed and the various criteria established for the particular conditions exercising in water.

With some ingenuity on the part of physiotherapists, classes can be conducted for a wide range of conditions exercising simultaneously. It is not necessary to have all participants suffering from a similar disorder. A wide range of techniques can be utilized and recreational activities introduced to increase the participation for the individual and their enjoyment.

THERAPEUTIC SWIMMING

In some countries hydrotherapy is considered to be a hydrotherapy treatment carried out in water by physiotherapists. When it comes to swimming there are those physiotherapists who see such activity as recreational and not their concern. The editor and authors of this book believe that swimming is an integral part of hydrotherapy programmes and forms part of the patients overall rehabilitation. As such it can be considered as therapeutic swimming and is best undertaken by the physiotherapist who has extensive training in movement and knows the pathology of disease. For physiotherapists who have also undertaken training in hydrotherapy techniques and in the recreational aspects of water activity, therapeutic swimming should certainly be their province.

Slade and Simmons-Grab (1987) suggest that therapeutic water programmes supervised by trained physiotherapists may be designed to cover exercise in water, instruction in appropriately amended swimming strokes and therapeutic recreational swimming. Involvement of personnel from other disciplines, such as swimming teachers who have trained in adapted aquatics through courses provided by tertiary institutions, is desirable.

There is little doubt that today water activity and swimming are favoured by the medical profession in treating a wide variety of conditions both medical and surgical. This is supported by the upsurge in the numbers of referrals for hydrotherapy, the suggestions made by doctors to their patients to swim to keep fit and the installation of an increasing number of pools. Swimming is a most useful activity (Kraus, 1973) because it can be so readily adapted to suit each individual's needs and capabilities—able bodied and disabled alike. This aspect of recreational water activity is an important part of the Halliwick method of swimming for the disabled (Reid Campion, 1985). The method is suitable for all but especially for the disabled of any age with any disability and any degree of that disability. In fact, the more severely disabled benefit considerably (Reid, 1975).

The buoyancy of the water diminishes the effects of gravity and thus reduces the stress on the joints. It also allows easier movement and where muscles are weak this is a distinct advantage. In water it is possible to perform movements, patterns of movement and feats which may be difficult or impossible on land (Grove, 1970; Campion, 1983). At the same time the impedance to movement due to the density of the liquid, the turbulent effects and the need to expend more energy to move in water facilitates the strengthening of muscles, increases range of motion and flexibility.

An important advantage, especially when considering functional training, is that the execution of exercises in water can be carried out in the erect position without strain due to the loss of weight in water. However, it is possible to exercise and swim in the horizontal without the need to gain the upright posture. Upthrust or buoyancy, and the support of water make movement easier and provides motivation to move more. This is important for enjoyment, happiness and morale.

Slade and Simmons-Grab (1987) suggest rehabilitation for many patients is a long-term process and the reality is that much of this can take place in therapeutic swimming programmes within the community. A considerable advantage for many swimmers however disabled is that they are able to find total independence in water. On land many disabled persons have to use some form of aid. In the medium of water the swimmer discards the wheelchair or other aids and can learn to control his own body in the water without resorting to flotation equipment or other devices. In most instances one such independence is gained it is possible for the disabled person to join with able bodied peers in a social activity and may also offer the opportunity to compete with their normal counterparts (Campion, 1983).

Experience has shown that the teaching of vertical and lateral rotational control, breathing and head control as advocated by the Halliwick method is valuable for everyone. When dealing with the head and spinal cord injured as well as with rheumatic, orthopaedic and other neurological conditions these skills are an essential part of the programme whether this is a hydrotherapeutic exercise programme or for therapeutic swimming. In this way the goals of general health and fitness as well as mobility and flexibility are achieved and when the patient is discharged from hospital may be maintained by participation in community programmes based on treatment schemes.

The selection of swimming strokes is vitally important. This means that not only must the physiotherapist understand the patient's condition and mobility in detail, but must also have knowledge of the muscle groups involved throughout the body for each individual. A strong stable trunk is essential from which the upper and lower limbs must work as they propel the body through the water. This suggests that throughout the rehabilitation programme the whole person should be treated and not just the affected part, so that ultimately the patient can use therapeutic swimming as a means of remaining fit.

As Slade and Simmons-Grab (1987) indicate such therapeutic water activity has considerable potential for rehabilitation for many differing disabilities, many severe. Such programmes give considerable help both physically and psychologically to the patients and to their families and friends, and permits integration into the more normal aspects of living. The physiotherapist's role in this type of activity is an essential one because of their training and knowledge of disabilities and mobility. They can give the appropriate exercise and swimming activity and thus avoid some of the potentially dangerous movements. If swimming is to be adapted to the needs of the individual and based on that person's mobility then this should be considered as therapeutic swimming. As in all training programmes suitable exercises are used to improve movement, strength and stamina and so these should be included in any therapeutic swimming programme.

Orientation to the water plays an important part in group therapeutic exercise programmes advocated by Slade and Simmons-Grab (1987). They suggest walking in various directions be used as a means of orientation and extend this to prone kicking for cardiovascular exercise. In Western Australia walking forwards, backwards and sideways would be used as a warm up and in some situations swimming laps might be used for the same purpose.

The teaching of mental adjustment and balance restoration, which in Western Australia is considered part of the orientation process, has been found essential to the orientation of patients whether entering the water for hydrotherapy or therapeutic swimming programmes. It ensures that the person's anxiety is lessened and that activity in water is undertaken with a greater degree of confidence and cooperation. The two factors, mental adjustment and balance restoration, are thus essential preliminaries to any programme (see p. 17).

Mental adjustment means that the swimmer appreciates the effects of buoyancy, turbulence, and the weight of water and has acquired a degree of breathing and head-control. *Balance restoration* involves teaching the swimmer both vertical and lateral rotational control and a combination of these rotations. A combination of these two rotations ensures that the swimmer is always able to recover to a safe breathing position.

A balanced floating position that can be controlled against all disturbing forces and the ability to regain the upright position ensures the swimmer will be safe in water. Once mentally adjusted and physically balanced the person is able to work effectively in the water and cooperate with the physiotherapist and cope with the demands of the programme. Learning swimming strokes requires balance, buoyancy, flotation and relaxation. The external and internal forces acting on a human body and the effects produced by these forces are studied when the biomechanics of stroking is undertaken. The greatest barrier to good stroking is tension, an internal resistance. If the swimmer has been taught the basic skills relating to breathing, head control and rotational control and is thus mentally adjusted to and physically balanced in water, swimming will come easily.

In all this, the swimmer will gain an understanding of body function, body awareness, spatial awareness particularly through the 'feel' of water and turbulence of which one is most aware at the distal parts of the limbs (Reid Campion, 1985). Harmonious movement is developed as it is easier to shift between contraction or relaxation of muscles (Myrenburg and Myrenburg, 1982).

Whatever the patient's condition there will be physical and psychological advantages accruing from a therapeutic water activity programme. These effects cover a wide range from kinaesthetic stimulation, cognitive sensorimotor patterns, improved circulation, the reduction of pain and muscle spasm, improved metabolism, re-education of muscle groups and improved range of motion. Morale and confidence are boosted by recreational activity; functional abilities are improved along with balance and coordination.

When therapeutic swimming takes place in the community benefits common to group activities occur. These include motivation and socialization. Since some therapeutic swimming would take place as a home programme or within the community, a means whereby the patient can move into the community again is provided; thus the patient can experience all the benefits brought about by such an action.

Breathing control is vital for good swimming and it has important effects on relaxation and thus aids balance (Reid Campion, 1985). Relaxation can be achieved by mental adjustment to the element of water; by the ability to regain and maintain a safe breathing position. With the other basic skills suggested previously the patient can participate in an activity which is a good method of keeping fit, improves endurance and stamina, produces a feeling of general well-being and provides social and psychological benefits that can be pursued throughout life.

REFERENCES

Bennett R.P. (1951). Water as a Medium for Therapeutic Exercise, *N.Y. St. J. Med.*, **51**, 513.

Bolton E., Goodwin D. (1979). *An Introduction to Pool Exercises*, Edinburgh: Churchill Livingstone.

Campion M. (1983). Water activity base on the Halliwick Method, In *Duffield's Exercise in Water*, 3rd edn. (Skinner A., Thomson A. eds). London: Baillière Tindall.

Cotton E., Kinsman R. (1983). *Conductive Education for Adult Hemiplegia*, Edinburgh: Churchill Livingstone.

Davis, B.C., Harrison, R.A. (1988). *Hydrotherapy in Practice*, Edinburgh: Churchill Livingstone.

Grove F. (1970). Aquatic therapy; a first real step to rehabilitation. *Journal of Health, Physical Education and Recreation. October*; 65.

Harris R., McInnes M. (1963). Exercises in water. In *Medical Hydrology* (Licht S. ed.) pp 207–17. New Haven: Elizabeth Licht.

Kamenetz, H.L. (1963). History of American spas and hydrotherapy, In *Medical Hydrology*, (Licht S. ed). New Haven: Elizabeth Licht Publisher.

Kraus R. (1973). *Therapeutic Recreation Service, Principles and Practice*, Philadelphia: W.B. Saunders Company.

Lowman, C.L., Roen, S.G. (1952). *Therapeutic Uses of Pools and Tanks*, pp 12, 69–70 Philadelphia: William B. Saunders.

Myrenburg K., Myrenburg M. (1982). *Watergymnastics*, Stockholm: Spänstituets Gymnastikförening.

Reid M.J. (1975). *Handling the Disabled Child in Water – an Introduction*, London Association of Chartered Paediatric Physiotherapists.

Reid Campion M. (1985). *Hydrotherapy in Paediatrics*, Oxford: Heinemann Medical Books.

Slade C., Simmons-Grab D. (1987). Therapeutic swimming as a community based programme. *Cognitive Rehabilitation*, **March/April**: 18–20.

Skinner A.T., Thomson A.M. eds (1983). *Duffield's Exercises in Water* 3rd edn. London: Baillière Tindall.

HYDROTHERAPY—A MEANS OF REHABILITATION

INTRODUCTION TO SECTION II

The following chapters cover neurological, neurosurgical, rheumatic, orthopaedic conditions and trauma attached to sports injuries. A study of the historical background to hydrotherapy shows that even in ancient times and down through the ages the value of water in the treatment of all the above mentioned conditions was recognized.

Hippocrates (c.460–375 BC) not only advocated the use of water for the treatment of a wide variety of diseases, but taught that it could be employed as a tonic and a sedative. Homer suggested that warm baths were efficacious in overcoming fatigue. More recently it has been said that water enhances the ability to feel (Bennett, 1951) and physiotherapists will readily see the advantage this has when treating patients suffering from neurological conditions. In the 5th century BC the Greeks recognized the essential nature of a pool as an adjunct to their sporting activities and the Romans followed in the footsteps of the Greeks. In this same century a Roman residing in Northern Africa used some modern concepts of physical treatment when he prescribed the use of natural waters, especially warm springs for paralysed patients as a means of restoration. He advocated swimming in the sea or warm springs 'initially with an inflated bladder attached to the paralysed part to reduce the effort required in swimming'.

The tide ebbed and flowed in ensuing centuries but by the 15th, 16th, and 17th centuries the use of water as a therapeutic measure was increasingly recognized. Sir John Floyer (1697) and John Wesley (1747) wrote about the value of water in the treatment of many diseases. The scientific background to hydrotherapy was promoted in the latter part of the 19th century and the early decades of the 20th century. Hydrotherapy as we know it today really began in the 1920s and major developments with specific techniques are of much more recent times.

The use of hydrotherapy in the treatment of rheumatic, orthopaedic and some neurological conditions is widely recognized, although the application of some techniques in neurological problems are questioned particularly in upper motor neuron lesions.

The advantages and/or disadvantages of treating the neuro-surgical patient in water varies from authority to authority, but it is hoped that some of the arguments may be laid to rest by the ensuing chapters and that physiotherapists will be encouraged to treat such patients in water and discover the value for themselves.

Sports injuries respond well to hydrotherapy, but sadly it is an area that has been neglected. Physiotherapists working in this field are aware of the benefits of the modality but fail to use water specifically allowing patients to pursue exercises in the medium that have come straight from the gymnasium which means that the unique advantages of water are not utilized to enhance the speedy recovery of these injuries. This section of the book provides interesting and exciting ways of utilizing water in the overall rehabilitation of many conditions.

Bennett R. L. (1951). Water as a medium for therapeutic exercise, *N.Y. St. J. Med.*, **51**, 513.

3

Hydrotherapy For The Neuro-surgical Patient

This chapter is based on the work done by the physiotherapy team in the neuro-surgical unit at Royal Perth (Rehabilitation) Hospital, Western Australia. This unit admits cases of brain trauma from causes such as motor vehicle accidents, motor cycle accidents, industrial and sporting accidents. These patients may or may not have required neuro-surgery. Additionally, the unit admits all cases of neuro-surgery for vascular complications and space-occupying lesions, such as arterio-venous malformations, aneurysms and tumours.

All cases admitted to the unit require rehabilitation. Each patient is reviewed by the physiotherapist and an appropriate rehabilitation programme is devised. Due to the extremes in conscious state of the patient case load catered for, from the comatosed patient to the ambulant patient, the physiotherapeutic care offered is accordingly tailored to suit. The programme offered covers respiratory physiotherapy, orthopaedic physiotherapy, physiotherapy in soft tissue injury, sensory bombardment and movement rehabilitation and cardio-vascular fitness. In the following chapter, the criteria for the choice of hydrotherapy as a treatment modality for the above mentioned cross-section of patients is delineated.

Problems faced by the neuro-surgical patient, in his attempt to regain normal or near normal function, are itemized. Each problem listed is explained and, where appropriate, treatment techniques are provided. It is important to bear in mind that each patient will have multiple problems and these must be addressed simultaneously if a beneficial outcome is to be achieved.

The exercises given in each section are not listed in order of progression, unless otherwise stated. The exercises exemplify the rationale of treatment and often the one exercise can be utilized to achieve a number of goals. Becoming familiar with some of the techniques, the reader should go on to formulating her own list of exercises using the same rationalization of treatment goals.

The chapter is divided into four areas:

• indications for hydrotherapy

- contra-indications to hydrotherapy
- untoward effects
- hints for success.

The introduction of the patient to water is vitally important. Consideration must be given to the dependency of the patient, size, weight, shape and density. The neuro-surgical patient can pose numerous problems in each of these areas. When a patient is totally dependent, two assistants may be needed to place the patient on the hoist. A physiotherapist or attendant should, as far as possible, be in the patient's line of vision or have a reassuring hand on the patient's shoulder. Where an increase in tone has altered the patient's shape, balancing the patient on the hoist satisfactorily can be brought about by the physiotherapist sitting alongside the patient on the hoist being lowered into the water with the patient.

Where a patient has poor or no head control, an inflatable collar is placed around the patient's neck and secured firmly. When the patient is floated off the hoist into the water, his head should rest on the physiotherapist's shoulder. The physiotherapist's hands should support the patient as low down the trunk as possible, using a backing hold in the horizontal position. If the patient is tall, a pelvic float may be required (Fig. 3.1).

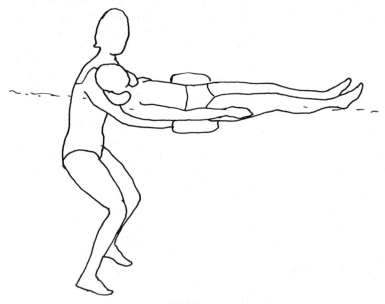

Fig. 3.1

INDICATIONS FOR HYDROTHERAPY

Hydrotherapy is indicated for the neuro-surgical patient where the desired goals are to:

- decrease tone
- stimulate movement
- retrain and stimulate righting reactions
- augment and increase the range of any weak movement
- retrain centralized, that is rotational, patterns of movement
- retrain reciprocal patterns of movement
- access functional movement patterns
- encourage and develop efficient breath control and voice production
- produce psychological effects
- treat any orthopaedic complications
- increase cardio-vascular fitness
- offer opportunities for recreation and socialization

To Decrease Tone

The reduction of tone may occur as a direct result of the warmth of the water. The support and the uniformity of stimulation provided by this medium help towards a further reduction of tone. The latter effect can be augmented by the use of techniques that utilize the vestibular connections in the central nervous system (CNS).

Research into the physiological effects of heat gives some clues as to the effects of heat on muscle tone. Fisher and Solomon (1965) indicate that the neck exteroceptors in the skin, when stimulated by warmth, show a diminution of gamma-fibre activity, which leads to decreased spindle excitability. Effects of general hyperthemia, on the reduction of tone, have been documented by Skinner and Thomson (1983). The simplest way to cause general hyperthermia is by immersion in water held at a temperature of 35°C (Franchimont *et al.*, 1983). This pool temperature has proved beneficial in attempts to reduce tone and this is borne out by the experience of the author in treating neuro-surgical patients and documented in the work of other physiotherapists (Harris, 1978).

When working with the head injured patient, in the water or on land, it must be remembered that the patient's thermo-regulatory ability is not as efficient as in the healthy individual. Much research has been done on the reflex increase in the gamma bias in the muscle spindle and an increase in tone can be achieved when core temperature falls by 0.4°C (Blatteis, 1960). It is of utmost importance that due consideration be given to the temperature of the water in the pool if the aim of treatment is the reduction of tone. The best response is obtained when pool temperature is maintained around 35°C, but not above when the beneficial effects tend to dissipate (Franchimont *et al.*, 1983).

The support offered by water and the consequent reduction/ elimination of the effects of gravity benefit both the physiotherapist and the patient. On land, the physiotherapist has to contend with the weight of the patient or the weight of a limb, where the patient is dependent. An average male patient may weigh 50–60 kg, which makes considerable demands on the physiotherapist. In any one day, the physiotherapist may have to treat up to 10 patients. This load can be reduced for the physiotherapist if treatment is carried out in the water by the judicious use of buoyancy and flotation, where the changes in position and shape of the patient can be achieved with minimal stress on the physiotherapist.

Activity on land requires the patient to contend with the forces of gravity acting on the affected and unaffected sides of the body. In attempting any movement, the patient has to cope with the uneven forces created by the contraction of muscles on the two sides of the body, the affected and unaffected side. From this background, patients are not only required to move through space, but also to maintain their balance. Tone is increased in proportion to the 'perceived effort'—as seen by the patient, being required to achieve the desired movement.

In the water, Archimedes' principle of relative density and Bougier's theorem of Metacentre (Reid Campion, 1985) can be utilized effectively to alleviate the above problem. The patient can be led to experience a sense of weightlessness and total support. The physiotherapist is then able to guide the patient through the required movement such that the patient's 'perceived effort' is decreased and tone is thereby reduced.

In attempting to use vestibular stimulation to reduce tone, the physiotherapist must be able to ensure a secure hold on the patient. This is affected by the altered shape of the patient and the distribution of the patient's body weight as a result of this altered shape. Using the principle of buoyancy and flotation, the physiotherapist is able to give the patient the required support only in water whilst ensuring an effective treatment. Slow rhythmical movements reduce tone whilst rapid movements increase tone. Slow rhythmical movements comprise all forms of swinging, rocking and rolling movements. Sullivan *et al.*, (1982) indicate that rotation around the longitudinal axis of the body aids in the reduction of spasticity.

Exercises to Decrease Tone

The reduction of tone may be brought about in the following ways:

1. ● Starting position: the patient lies in front of the physiotherapist, who uses a backing hold in the horizontal position.
   ● Technique: the physiotherapist walks slowly backwards. Initially, the patient is taken backwards through the water in a straight line. Later, the physiotherapist, by walking in a 'lazy s' shaped path, allows lateral trunk flexion to occur.
   ● Patient appreciation: the patient appreciates the sensory stimulation provided by the warmth and the pressure of the water, and the movement of the hips and lower limbs on the trunk.
2. ● Starting position: as above.
   ● Technique: as the physiotherapist walks backwards and sways the patient from side to side, the physiotherapist raises the hip first on one side and then the other at the end of the swing, thereby incorporating some rotation.
   ● Patient appreciation: the patient feels the sensory stimulation provided by the water — the warmth and pressure — as well as the movement of the hips and lower limbs on the trunk, coupled with trunk rotation.
3. ● Starting position: the patient is in supine lying facing the physiotherapist, who has the patient's legs on either side of the physiotherapist's waist and her hands under the patient's hips. The patient's head is supported by an inflatable neck collar.
   ● Technique: the physiotherapist moves the patient slowly in an arc. The arc is progressively widened (Fig. 3.2).
   ● Patient appreciation: the patient appreciates the sensory stimulation of the warmth and pressure of the water, the movement of the head and trunk on the hips and stimulation of the vestibular-ocular system (Herman, 1982).

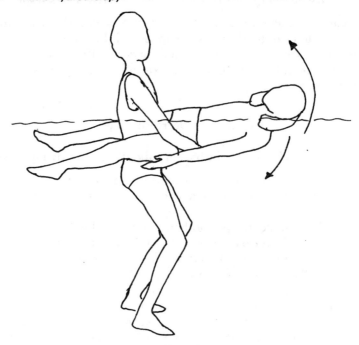

Fig. 3.2

4. ● Starting position: the patient is held curled up in a ball
   sideways on to the physiotherapist. The patient's knees
   are flexed up against the chest, with the patient's hands
   around the knees, where possible (see Fig. 3.3). The
   physiotherapist holds the patient with one arm placed
   around the patient's back at waist level, the other hand
   holds the patient's legs in flexion. The depth at which the
   activity takes place should be such that the greater part of
   the patient's weight is supported by the water.
   ● Technique: the therapist, by rhythmically and slowly
   moving her body laterally in a rocking motion, causes a
   forward and backward movement of the patient's body.
   Initially, a small amplitude displacement of the patient's
   head is aimed for.
   ● Patient appreciation: the patient appreciates the movement of the head and neck on the trunk and vestibular
   stimulation.

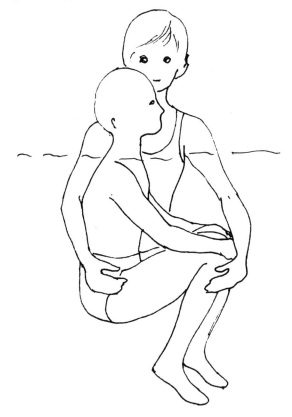

To Stimulate Movement

It is necessary to stimulate the return of movement in the severely disabled patient who invariably has very little in the way of voluntary movement. At this stage of the patient's recovery, there is considerable sensory deprivation and the patient thus has very little desire to move. The patient may not know how to move.

It is known that thermal information is carried via collateral pathways from the spinothalamic and lemniscal tracts to the mid-brain and the reticular formation in the brainstem. This information is then carried along neural pathways from the latter areas to the hypothalamic and pre-optic areas (Lee and Warren, 1978). The function of the reticular formation is to stimulate the cortex to wakefulness. Therefore, heat, by stimulating the neural receptors in the skin (Wadsworth and Chanmugam, 1983) and its connections to the reticular formation along with vestibular information, which also has connections in the reticular formation, helps maintain a state of alertness in the patient.

Any movement of the head in space will cause varying degrees of vestibular stimulation. The vestibular system has connections with the reticular formation and the cerebellum. The latter is an important centre, together with the thalamus and mid-brain in the control of muscular tone. Herman (1982) in his research postulates that the prerequisite of peripheral movement is mid-line structure stability and visual stability, in particular the vestibular-ocular reflex. The latter reflex is brought into operation when the head is moved in space in relation to a stationary object.

The above explanations allow the basis for the formulation of exercises that will result in the stimulation and establishment of tone and movement. Where the eyes go, the head follows and so the body. Where movement is already present, however little, further movement may be produced as a result of stimulation overflow and recruitment of motor neurons. The latter is the basis for some of the proprioceptive neuro-muscular facilitation (PNF) techniques.

5. ● Starting position: the patient is in the horizontal supine float position with his lower limbs on either side of the physiotherapist's waist. The physiotherapist's hands support the patient as high up the back as possible (Fig. 3.2).
   ● Technique: the patient is rotated to allow the cheek on that side to touch the water, whilst being given instruction to turn the head away. In the initial stages, the whole pattern can be done passively by the physiotherapist. At first, displacement is small, but is progressively allowed to get larger.
   ● Patient appreciation: the patient appreciates vestibular stimulation and head on body turning.

Techniques numbered (1) to (5) could be introductory lessons before attempting techniques (6), (7) and (8).

6. ● Starting position: the physiotherapist holds the patient as in the previous technique, except that the hands holding the patient support the hips.
   ● Technique: this technique is a progression on the previous one. The physiotherapist displaces the patient's hips from side to side with an anterior/posterior movement. The

patient is instructed not to allow any movement to occur, initially. As the range of displacement is increased, the patient is instructed to return head and trunk to midline.

- Patient appreciation: the patient appreciates vestibular stimulation; in addition there is static work for the trunk extensors, which is progressed to active head and trunk extension and rotation.

7. • Starting position: the patient is held in the horizontal supine float position with the lower limbs astride the physiotherapist's waist (Fig. 3.2). If the patient is tall or heavy, a pelvic float may also be required.

- Technique: the patient is moved in an arc in one direction only. When the appropriate momentum has been gained, the physiotherapist stops the movement abruptly. The patient's trunk will be carried on passively in the line of movement till all momentum is dissipated.

- Patient appreciation: the patient appreciates vestibular stimulation, as well as lateral flexion of the trunk.

8. • Starting position: the starting position is the same as that in technique seven (Fig. 3.2).

- Technique: the patient is instructed to touch the ipsilateral knee with the hand on the side of the direction of movement. For example, if the patient is being moved to the right, the instruction is to touch the right knee with the right hand. This technique is first performed to the stronger side.

- Patient appreciation: the patient appreciates vestibular stimulation and lateral flexion of the trunk, which is voluntary and assisted. The patient has had to work from the area of turbulence or drag effect and against bow wave, both of which impede the movement.

9. • Starting position: the patient is held in the horizontal supine float position with the lower limbs astride the physiotherapist's waist (Fig. 3.2).

- Technique: the patient is moved in an arc to the affected side (Fig. 3.4). When the physiotherapist stops the movement of the patient's body through the water, the patient is instructed not to let the water cause lateral flexion of the body. This will bring about contraction of the trunk flexors of the unaffected side. When the patient has learnt the sequence, the movement can be taken to the unaffected side.

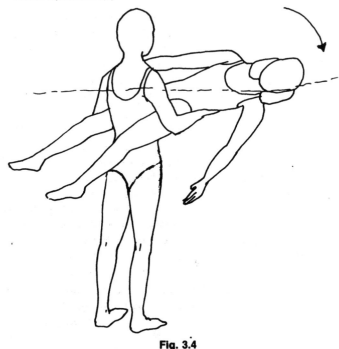

Fig. 3.4

- Patient appreciation: the patient appreciates the static muscle work of the trunk side flexors on the affected side.
10. ● Starting position: the patient is supported by neck and pelvic floats and is in the horizontal supine float position facing away from the physiotherapist. The unaffected or least affected leg is placed in a ring float with the appropriate amount of air in it, so that the leg is just floated to the surface. The affected leg is allowed to sink in the water. The physiotherapist supports the patient as required.
- Technique: the patient is instructed to push the ankle float ring under the water.
- Patient appreciation: the patient appreciates the 'movement' of the affected leg to the surface. The patient is subsequently instructed to augment the movement of the affected limb so that it moves to the surface quickly.

Retrain and Stimulate Righting Reactions

The ability of the body to right itself is seemingly dependent on tone. When hypotonus is present, for example, when there is damage to the cerebellum, few, if any, righting reactions persist. The presence of hypertonus, on the other hand, dampens the body's ability to utilize stepping, propping and righting reactions. These protective mechanisms are difficult to retrain on land as they are the means by which the unsupported body gains stability. It is extremely difficult to give adult patients enough support, to enable them to have the confidence to relearn these antigravity reactions.

In the correct depth of water, with appropriate support from the physiotherapist, the patient can be given the required feeling of support and security. This is the base from which the patient can be taught the destabilizing effects of limb movements on the body and the appropriate counter-measures to regain stability. The techniques described from (1) to (9) above, utilize head and trunk righting and can be used to retrain and stimulate righting reactions.

11. ● Starting position: the patient is facing the physiotherapist in a stride sitting position on the latter's lap. The physiotherapist maintains a stable 'sitting' position, one hand being taken under the patient's arm and placed in the thoraco-lumbar area, whilst the other hand is placed in the occipital and neck area. The patient's upper limbs are placed on the physiotherapist's shoulders. This is the ideal position for the patient's arms and hands, but is not always easy to achieve and maintain (Fig. 3.5).
    ● Technique: the patient is instructed to keep the face level with that of the physiotherapist, who shifts her weight from one leg to the other. Thus, the patient's hip and trunk are displaced laterally.
    ● Patient appreciation: the patient appreciates the head and trunk righting brought about by this technique.
12. ● Starting position: the patient is in horizontal supine float lying, supported by neck and hip floats and facing away from the physiotherapist, who stands close to the patient's head supporting the patient in the lower thoracic region with both hands (Fig. 3.6).
    ● Technique: the patient is asked to slowly lift one arm out of the water close to the side of the body. Such action will cause the body to roll to the side on which the arm is

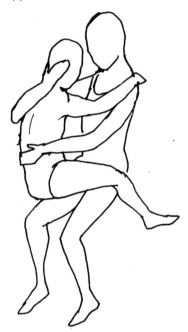

Fig. 3.5

lifted. As the trunk begins to rotate, the patient is
instructed to turn the head away from the side rolling
under and drop the shoulder into the water on the side to
which the head is turned. Initially, assistance is given as
needed, but as the patient masters the technique the
physiotherapist's support is slowly withdrawn.

- Patient appreciation: the patient appreciates the effects of
  limb movement on the stability of the body. Awareness of
  the righting reactions to counter the destabilization of the
  body and appreciation of static work for the trunk
  muscles.

13. - Starting position: the patient assumes a stable, sitting
     position in the water. This position, ideally, requires that
     there is a right angle at hips, knees and ankles, the feet
     being hip width apart, the shoulders under the water, the
     arms stretched forwards and the trunk upright. The phy-
     siotherapist adopts a position behind the patient, support-
     ing the patient's hips to stabilize these joints (Fig. 3.7).

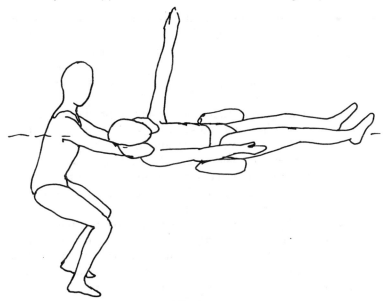

Fig. 3.6

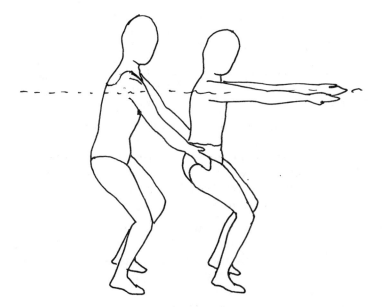

Fig. 3.7

- Technique: the patient is instructed to stretch the fingers as far forwards as possible. When the physiotherapist feels the patient is about to fall forwards, the patient is instructed to sit lower in the water, at the same time the physiotherapist applies pressure downwards on the patient's hips.
- Patient appreciation: the patient appreciates the static work of the trunk muscles, as well as the destabilizing effect of limb movement and the activity required to regain balance when the body is falling forward.

14.
- Starting position: the patient is in a stable sitting position as indicated in technique (13), and the physiotherapist maintains the same stable stance.
- Technique: the patient is instructed to lower the arms into the water, thus causing the patient to disturb the balanced position. As the physiotherapist feels the patient's balance is disturbed, the patient is instructed to take the head forward and reach as far forward as possible with the fingers. Frequently, it is helpful to have the patient reach towards a visual target, for example, the side of the pool.
- Patient appreciation: the patient appreciates the contraction of the head and trunk flexor muscles, as well as the destabilizing effect brought about by limb movement and the activity required to regain balance, when the body is moved backwards in relation to the base of support.

Once the patient has some knowledge of maintaining the balance of the body against forward and backward displacement, the techniques can be progressed in various ways:

- the patient is instructed to look in various directions, up and down and side to side.
- the patient is instructed to lower one arm and move it forward and backwards in the water.
- the patient is instructed to move both arms in the water.
- the patient is instructed to flex one leg up.

Techniques (12), (13) and (14) utilize the principles of relative density, turbulence and metacentre (Reid Campion, 1985). These techniques are particularly useful for patients who show ataxic signs. It gives the patient a concept of mid-line structure stability whilst moving peripheral structures. It also allows active relearning of righting reactions whilst in a stable upright position.

Augment and Increase the Range of any Weak Movements

With the patient in a stable position, judicious positioning of the limbs or angle of movement can augment and increase the range of any weak movement. This can be equally applied to upper motor neuron type paralysis, as well as lower motor neuron types of muscular weakness.

In central nervous system lesions, the increased effort to move the limb against gravity causes further increases in tone. In water, by allowing buoyancy to assist, the weak movement is allowed to move through a greater range than would otherwise have been possible. In doing so, a concomitant increase in tone as a result of co-contraction or associated reactions can be diminished.

15. ● Starting position: the patient assumes a stable sitting position on the physiotherapist's lap, facing away from the physiotherapist who maintains a stabilizing hold on the patient's hips. As an alternative, the patient can be supported by neck and pelvic floats in a horizontal supine float position.
    ● Technique: the affected limb or more affected limb is pushed passively and rapidly into the water. The upthrust effect of water will ensure that the limb returns to the surface. This action is repeated a number of times. The patient is then instructed to assist in the return of the limb to the surface of the water.
    ● Patient appreciation: the patient becomes aware of the effect of upthrust or buoyancy of the water and once appreciation of the upward movement of the limb has taken place, the patient, when asked to assist the movement, conceptualizes the gradual muscle strength required to move the limb.
16. ● Starting position: the patient is in the horizontal supine float position or in supported side lying, for example, on a plinth in the water. Flotation equipment is applied to the limb.
    ● Technique: all the anatomical movements of the limbs can be practised, for example, in the side lying position; upper and lower limb flexion and extension movements can be attempted.
    ● Patient appreciation: the patient appreciates movement practised through as large a range as possible. Such

movements are comparable to exercises done in sling suspension on land.

17. ● Starting position: the patient is placed in the standing position in a depth of water that is at the level of the xiphisternum. Depending on the degree of dependence of the patient, one or two physiotherapists may be required to support the patient whose arms are placed around the physiotherapists' shoulders.

● Technique: walking practice is encouraged and lateral weight shift is initiated by the physiotherapists.

● Patient appreciation: in the water, with minimal effort and the assistance of buoyancy, extensor tone can be over-ridden and leg flexion is then possible, whereas, on land, the standing position can cause an increase in extensor tone to the extent that the patient is unable to flex the limb against the strength of the extensor tone. Therefore, practising ambulation in the pool will prove beneficial.

Retain Centralized (rotational) Pattern of Movement

Lateralizing motor deficits result in abnormal posture. Any peripheral limb or head movement occurring from this central abnormal trunk posture will be inefficient and of poor quality. Control of trunk patterns of movement can only be learnt in a position where the effect of gravity is neutralized. Water offers this ideal medium.

A common problem encountered in the neuro-surgical patient is the lack of shoulder and hip girdle movement and a paucity of trunk rotation. This is often seen in the 'robot' walking pattern, where the patient has very little arm swing, head turning, trunk rotation and 'ambles' along with a 'waddling' gait.

18. ● Starting position: the patient is in supine lying at a right angle and to one side of the physiotherapist, who supports the patient with the arm on the side to which the patient is lying. The physiotherapist's arm is at the level of the inferior angle of the scapulae.

● Technique: to create a roll through 360° in front of the physiotherapist, the patient is instructed to turn the head towards the physiotherapist and to bring the outer arm and leg across the body. The physiotherapist's free arm acts as a guide and support for the patient's arm as it comes across and may facilitate the rolling action. At the completion of the roll, the patient will be in the same starting position, but on the opposite side of the physiotherapist (Reid Campion, p. 57, 1985) (Fig. 3.8).

- Patient appreciation: the patient will appreciate marked vestibular stimulation along with head control, trunk rotation and body righting.

19. - Starting position: the patient is in the horizontal supine float lying position with the physiotherapist standing between the legs at the level of the patient's knees and supporting the patient with the hands placed as high up the patient's back as possible (Fig. 3.2).

- Technique: the patient is instructed to come up to sitting, initiating the movement with the head and reaching forward with the hands, which are placed on the physiotherapist's shoulders. To facilitate the forward movement, the physiotherapist must 'sit' down in the water as the patient comes up to the sitting position astride the physiotherapist's knee (Fig. 3.5). As the patient returns to the starting position, the head must control the movement of the body back into the lying position.

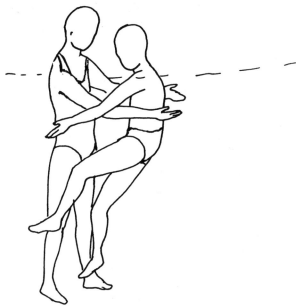

Fig. 3.8

● Patient appreciation: the patient becomes aware of the need for head control in initiating and controlling movement. Additionally, trunk flexion and the achievement of a functional movement from lying to sitting will be appreciated.

Retrain Reciprocal Pattern Movement

Midline structure stability provides the basis of limb movement as reciprocal patterns of movement provide the basis of functional patterns of locomotion. Reciprocal limb movements are affected by minimal changes in tone. If the patient is well supported and the limbs allowed to move freely, the patient is able to concentrate solely on coordinating the movement and not on the effort of moving. Rhythm contributes to the smoothness in the execution of any movement pattern. This is an important concept to teach the patient when reciprocal movements are being practised.

20. ● Starting position: the patient is in the horizontal supine float position supported by neck and pelvic floats. The physiotherapist assumes a position where the patient can be assisted maximally. This may be at the patient's head to steady the patient, if necessary, but the head itself should never be held, since this destroys the patient's last opportunity to control the body and lower limbs (Reid Campion, 1985). The physiotherapist may find it an advantage to stand by the patient's feet and guide the movement from that position.
    ● Technique: the patient is instructed to flex and extend each of the lower limbs in turn. To ensure that the limb remains in contact with the water, the movement is done with external rotation of the hip. The patient is encouraged to maintain a smooth movement pattern by counting to four for each cycle of movement.
    ● Patient appreciation: the patient becomes aware of coordination of the limbs, learns control of speed of movement and rhythm, so vital in neurological conditions.
21. ● Starting position: the patient is in the supine floating position as in technique (20). The physiotherapist stands behind the patient's head supporting the patient underneath the back at the level of the patient's waist.

- Technique: the patient is instructed to flex the leg in abduction and external rotation whilst taking the ipsilateral arm down to the knee, that is, for example, right hand to right knee. The patient will not roll if the contralateral arm and leg are held in extension.
- Patient appreciation: the patient will appreciate the movement of side flexion combined with coordination of the head, trunk and limbs. Body image and awareness of body parts will be enhanced.

22.
- Starting position: as in technique (20). The physiotherapist may stand at either the patient's head or feet. If standing at the head, support is provided underneath the patient's waist. However, if standing at the patient's feet, the hold is on the lateral side of the patient's ankles.
- Technique: the patient is instructed by the physiotherapist to abduct and then adduct the legs. It may be necessary to guide the movements of abduction and adduction when the position of the physiotherapist would be at the patient's feet.
- A rhythmic counting is essential in the early stages until the patient has mastered the movement and can take over the counting. Once the movements of the legs have been mastered, abduction and adduction of the arms should be incorporated. Initially, the arms should move in the same direction as the legs. Later, the patient should be encouraged to move the upper and lower limbs in opposite directions. Rhythmical movement must be obtained at all times. In this manner, the patient can learn to propel the body through the water.
- Patient appreciation: the patient appreciates coordination of all four limbs, concentration, movement disassociation and independent mobility in the water.

23.
- Starting position: the patient is placed in the prone horizontal float position supported by a pelvic float and with the hands on the physiotherapist's shoulders. Alternatively, the hands may be placed on an air ring.
- Technique: the patient is instructed to maintain extension at the knees and perform 'straight' kicks.
- Patient appreciation: the patient becomes aware of increasing strength in the neck, trunk and limb extensor muscle groups and lower limb coordination.

Access Functional Movement Patterns

All head injured patients have problems with new learning, to a greater or lesser extent. This problem is augmented in those patients with perceptual deficits, such as dyspraxia, decreased spatial awareness and decreased body image.

The dyspraxic patient will have great difficulty in planning and sequencing a set of exercise programmes, but may produce the desired movement when the exercise is practised as a functional movement pattern. This is exemplified by the patient who has great difficulty in coordinating arm swing whilst walking, but is able to coordinate all four limbs when swimming. This is especially evident in those patients who enjoyed swimming prior to the hospitalization. It is advisable to provide a float initially, so that the patient is not faced with failure at the first attempt.

24. ● Starting position: the patient is placed in the horizontal supine float position facing away from the physiotherapist, who supports the patient's body underneath the back at waist level with the patient's head resting on the physiotherapist's shoulder or close to the shoulder (Fig. 3.9a).

    ● Technique: the patient is instructed to flex both legs towards the chest, to bring the head, shoulders and arms forward and come to the sitting position. The patient is also instructed to blow out strongly as the head comes forward. Such action assists the forward movement of the head (Figs. 3.9b, 3.9c).

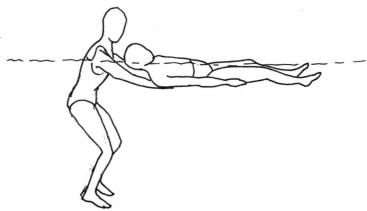

Fig. 3.9a

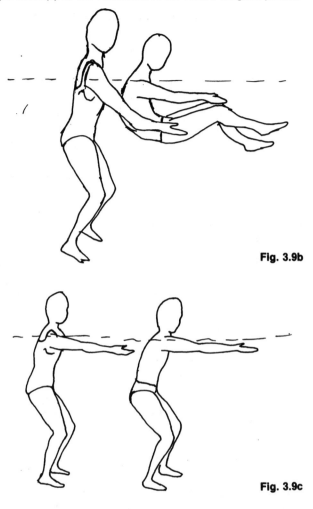

Fig. 3.9b

Fig. 3.9c

To return to the starting position, the patient is instructed to bring the legs towards the chest, place the head and shoulders back slowly and then straighten the legs.

The physiotherapist initially assists the patient to gain the sitting position. Gradually, such assistance is withdrawn so that the patient is finally able to accomplish the movement independently.

Balancing in the sitting position requires fine adjustments of the head, arms and hands with precise balance of the head on the spine. Turbulence judiciously and appropriately placed around the patient develops balance co-ordination to a greater degree once the patient is able to perform the lying to sitting action correctly and stabilize the body in the sitting position.

- Patient appreciation: the patient becomes aware of how to achieve functional movement pattern of getting from lying to sitting in water. This may carry over on to land; however, it must be realized that the pattern for land will differ in some ways from that in water.

There is increasing awareness of a developing range of movements of head, trunk and lower limb flexion, which are involved in vertical rotation control (Reid Campion, 1985).

Due to the support afforded by the water, walking practice is made easier for the physiotherapist and the patient. This support, the relaxation of tone, the assistance provided to movement by buoyancy and the decreased effort required to move limbs, will often allow a patient hampered by a strong positive supporting reaction on land to achieve movement in the water.

It is usually inadvisable to take a confused, restless and mobile patient into the water. Where a patient is restless and dependent, the restlessness can be directed to produce movement in the water with the use of appropriate flotation equipment and under the strict supervision of a physiotherapist, on a one-to-one basis with the patient. For the patient who is confused, but compliant and has enjoyed swimming prior to the accident, hydrotherapy is an ideal situation to start the introduction of a structured programme. The patient is allowed to move or swim by whatever means possible. The physiotherapist should be quick to observe the effect of altered body shape and provide appropriate support. Due to residual hemiparesis, a patient attempting to swim may find the affected side lagging in the water and thereby causing his body to roll. Providing the patient with a limb or trunk float or encouraging the patient to use an inflated rubber ring, may give the stability he needs. Encouraged by the success of his effort, the patient will then persist with this exercise.

By pacing the patient while the latter is 'swimming', allows the physiotherapist to slowly encourage the patient to concentrate on one activity. Aerobic activity is aided and this in turn helps the patient to concentrate. An exercise programme such as mat exercises will have no meaning to a confused patient, and their insistence will only encourage increasing levels of frustration for the patient. The sedative effects of heat and hydrotherapy on the restless patient have been documented by Wilson and Kasch (1963) and Kraus (1973).

Encourage and Develop an Efficient Breath Control and Voice Production

Voice production is dependent on good breathing patterns. Many patients who are mute or have poor phonation because of their head injury, have benefited from hydrotherapy conducted in collaboration with the speech pathologist (this is the term used in Australia for a speech therapist).

Briefly, efficient breath control and phonation is hampered by the increase in tone in the muscles of the neck and abdomen. This tone can effectively splint the expansion of the rib cage and diaphragmatic excursion required to produce effective breath control. In the water, emphasis is placed on total relaxation. This is obtained, in the horizontal supine float position, by the use of floats which provide total support to the arms, legs, trunk, neck and head. The relaxation achieved can be utilized to teach the patient proper use of the abdominal musculature to produce and control the rate and length of inspiration and expiration. The speech pathologist's participation is vital, preferably in the pool alongside the physiotherapist, to ensure that normal phonatory patterns and speech are successfully re-established.

Hydrotherapy encourages movement and play. Both can be used to facilitate and guide patients to produce voice and speech as part of their exercise programme. The speech pathologist should be encouraged to participate and contribute to this activity in the water.

The strength of oral musculature has bearing on both speech and effective feeding. To strengthen these muscles, blowing activities should be encouraged. Such activities include blowing bubbles in the water and also blowing lightweight plastic objects across the surface of the water.

Produce Psychological Effects

Whatever the style and however many floats it takes, the disabled patient gets enjoyment from moving through the water under his own volition. This allows the patient a sense of achievement and freedom and helps reinforce a positive attitude necessary for any long-term rehabilitation.

Hydrotherapy is a welcome break from routine for those patients who enjoy the water. When improvement is measured in months, patients enjoy the change of medium. Most people associate the pool with recreation, relaxation and enjoyment and therefore readily accept working in the water.

Treat any Orthopaedic Complication

The treatment of orthopaedic complications by hydrotherapy is covered in another chapter. The force of trauma that produces a head injury may also produce fractured limbs and/or spine.

When a patient is initially out of a plaster cast, joint stiffness causes pain and thus a reluctance to move the affected limb. This, in turn leads to increased joint stiffness and further pain. The warmth of the water relieves joint stiffness (Wadsworth and Chanmugam, 1983) and may decrease the perception of pain. In the case of a patient who has suffered a fracture of the tibia and fibula, when the plaster of paris cast is removed the attention is centred on the stiff joint—the knee and ankle. This will cause a stronger perception of pain, largely as a result of the expectation of pain and stiffness. Instead of focusing on knee flexion exercises, the physiotherapist should choose movement patterns that will involve knee flexion, such as technique (24), which provides a means of obtaining the desired increase in the range of the knee movement combined with total trunk patterns of movement (vertical rotation).

Head injured patients who are expected to grade the degree of weight bearing on the affected joint, especially when they have associated paralysis, can be helped by practising ambulation in the water. Depending on the depth of water chosen, the weight on the limb can be accurately monitored in terms of weight bearing of total body weight (Harrison and Bulstrode, 1987).

For patients with oedematous limbs, exercising in the deeper end of the pool will help decrease the swelling in the limbs in accordance with Pascal's Law (Reid Campion, 1985).

To Increase Cardio-vascular Fitness

A return to the demands of the patient's previous employment is unlikely where the patient has undergone neuro-surgery as the patient's medical condition compromises fitness. All patients expecting to return to work should be given a programme of cardio-vascular fitness training. Energy requirements to move in water are far greater than in air according to the work of Froude and Zahm (Reid Campion, 1985). Supervising a cardio-vascular fitness programme in the hydrotherapy pool is less time-consuming than on the land. The patient entering the pool for cardio-vascular fitness training will find a pool temperature of 35°C very exhausting; a venue with a lower pool temperature will have to be considered for this type of programme.

Opportunities for Recreation and Socialization

The severely disabled patient who finds independent movement difficult on land, may achieve such mobility in the water. The properties of water provide a medium where freedom of movement can be obtained.

By providing appropriate flotation equipment, the physiotherapist can teach the patient to utilize whatever mobility, that has been regained, to move through the water. The patient's shape and/or density will have been affected by the injury and this must be carefully assessed prior to using flotation equipment. Wherever possible, such equipment should be kept to a minimum, and the ideal is that the patient should be able to move through the water without any support, if total independence is to be gained.

A patient confined to a wheelchair, due to involuntary movements, will demonstrate a considerable diminution of the ataxic or choreoathetoid movements once in the water, provided the strokes are adapted to keep the limbs under the water. One such patient, despite the presence of severe choreoathetoid, ataxic and occasional ballistic movement as a result of a head injury, was taught to swim. He was initially taught relaxation, breath control and coordination. Selective strengthening of the extensor muscles was then implemented. This was followed by the retraining of rotational movement patterns. The patient was then taught swimming strokes. He now enjoys swimming, totally submerged. The breaststroke action used is totally coordinated whilst under the water, but any work on the surface is noticeably less coordinated.

Recreational activities, on land, require modification of equipment and able bodied helpers. In the water, an efficient assessment of the patient's ability and quality of movement by the physiotherapist is all that is needed to implement a similar programme.

Recreational programmes can be developed to cater for group activities. Neuro-surgical patients, especially the head injured, are often socially isolated by a motor, perceptual or behavioural problem. Working in a group helps the patient learn social skills necessary for integration into the mainstream of society.

CONTRA-INDICATIONS

- Some problems experienced by the neuro-surgical patient contra-indicate hydrotherapy as a treatment modality. When a diagnosis of fractured base of skull is made, it is important to seek the neurosurgeon's opinion prior to instituting a hydrotherapy programme. A fracture in the base of the skull points to possible communication into the meninges. If the patient inhales water, it is possible for water borne infection to communicate with the brain, giving rise to meningitis.
- Patients incontinent of bowel and bladder are not taken into the pool. The latter problem in male patients is easily overcome. Most dependent patients establish a routine of bladder and bowel continence spontaneously. This allows a hydrotherapy programme to be undertaken during the patient's 'dry periods'.
- The effect of the heat of the hydrotherapy pool on a patient with high blood pressure, especially if the latter is a result of a head injury, and on unclipped aneurysm, is unknown. These patients are not taken into the pool for a hydrotherapy programme.
- The following conditions exclude the affected patients from the pool:
  1 Methicillin resistant *Staphylococcus aureus*, diarrhoea or non diarrhoeal gastrointestinal infections, hepatitis A, non A non B hepatitis, vesicular skin conditions and patients with open or weeping lesions who are known or suspected to be carriers of blood borne diseases, e.g. hepatitis B or HIV.
  2 There is no reason to exclude patients with urinary tract infections from the pool as most of these infections are caused

by normal bowel organisms that do not pose any threat to other people.

UNTOWARD EFFECTS

Some patients may have adverse reactions after hydrotherapy sessions and it is important to take note of these:

- patients may exhibit an increase in tone. If this tone increase is a consistent feature after the 2nd or 3rd session, hydrotherapy should cease and may be re-introduced at a later date.
- some patients take on a 'hot flushed' look—this usually points to a physiological inability to cope with the heat and hydrotherapy is discontinued for a while.
- patients on sedative drugs to control restlessness may appear extremely lethargic and tired after a pool session.
- patients with very low blood pressure should be monitored closely. Their blood pressure before and after sessions should be taken.
- due to the nature of the patients' dependence, the patients are unable to communicate simple problems, like water being retained in the ear. It is important to ensure that the nursing staff look into this. Due to their debilitation, these patients are prone to persistent ear infections.

HINTS FOR SUCCESS

To be successful in treating a neuro-surgical patient in water, a few guidelines should be followed:

- where hydrotherapy is being used as a treatment modality and not as a recreational facility, treatment should always be on a one-to-one basis. Where group activity is involved in the treatment programme, the one-to-one basis operates within the group.
- treatment should be goal oriented. Having assessed the patient and analysed the main problems, the physiotherapist should develop an exercise programme that will achieve specific results.
- hydrotherapy should not be abandoned as a treatment modality if no success is initially forthcoming. The programme can be re-introduced at a later date for such a patient.

- where availability of trained assistants is a problem, family members can be trained to assist. This gives the family a sense of participation in the patient's recovery process. Being a part of the patient's programme is important to family members, as it helps them in their effort to come to terms with the tragedy that has occurred.
- introduce games towards the end of each session and allow group participation when possible.

REFERENCES

Blatteis C.M. (1960). Afferent stimulation of shivering. *American Journal of Physiology*, **199**, 698.

Fisher E., Solomon S. (1965). Physiological response to heat and cold. In (Licht S., Kamenetz H. L. eds.) *Therapeutic Heat and Cold*, pp. 126–169. Baltimore: Waverley Press.

Franchimont, P., Juchmes J., Lecomte J. (1983). Hydrotherapy—Mechanisms and Indications. *Pharmacology Therapeutics*, **20**, 79–93.

Harris, S.R. (1978). Neurodevelopmental treatment approach for teaching swimming to cerebral palsied children. *Physical Therapy*, **58**, 979–983.

Harrison, R., Bulstrode S. (1987). Percentage Weight Bearing During Partial Immersion in the Hydrotherapy Pool. *Physiotherapy Practice*, **3**, pp. 60–63.

Herman R. (1982). Functional Recovery in the Visual and Vestibular Pathways. *Int. Rehab. Med.*, **4**, pp. 173–176.

Kraus R. (1973). Therapeutic Recreation Services – Principles and Practices. Philadelphia: W.B. Saunders.

Lee J.M., Warren M.P. (1978). Cold Therapy in Rehabilitation. London: Bell & Hyman.

Reid Campion M. (1985). *Hydrotherapy in Paediatrics*. Oxford: Heinemann Medical Books Ltd.

Skinner, A.T., Thomson, A.M. (1983). Duffield's Exercise in Water. London: Baillière, Tindall.

Sullivan P.E., Markos, P.D., Minor M.A.D. (1982). An Integrated Approach to Therapeutic Exercise: Theory and Clinical Application. Reston, Va: Reston Pub. Co.

Wadsworth J., Chanmugam A.P.P. (1983). Electrophysical Agents in Physiotherapy, 2nd edn., Marrickville, N.S.W.: Science Press.

Wilson I.H., Kasch F.W. (1963). Medical Aspects of Swimming. In *Medical Hydrology* (Licht S. ed.) Newhaven: Elizabeth Licht Publisher.

RECOMMENDED READING

Euler, C.V., Soderberg, U. (1956). The Relation Between Gamma Motor Activity and the Electroencephalogram. *Experientia*, 12, pp. 278–279.

Harrison, R., Bulstrode, S. (1987). Percentage Weight Bearing During Partial Immersion in the Hydrotherapy Pool. *Physiotherapy Practice*, Vol. 3, pp. 60–63.

Herman, R. (1982). A Therapeutic Approach Based on Theories of Motor Control. *Int. Rehab. Med.*, 4, pp. 185–189.

Herman, R. (1982). Functional Recovery in the Visual and Vestibular Pathways. *Int. Rehab. Med.*, 4, pp. 173–173.

Ito Masae (1972). Neural Design of the Cerebellar Motor Control System. *Brain Research*, 40, pp. 81–84.

Reid Campion (1985). Hydrotherapy in Paediatrics. Oxford: Heinemann Medical Books.

Sullivan, P.E., Markos, P.D., Minor, M.A.D. (1982). An Integrated Approach to Therapeutic Exercise: Theory and Clinical Application. Reston, Va: Reston Pub. Co.

Wadsworth, H. and Chanmugan, A.P.P. (1983). Electrophysical Agents in Physiotherapy, 2nd Ed., Marrickville, N.S.W: Science Press.

ACKNOWLEDGEMENTS

Margaret Reid Campion—whose training and guidance has formed the basis of the treatment of neuro-surgical patients in hydrotherapy. My thanks to Margaret for allowing the liberal use of exercises and drawings from her book.

Serena Pearce and other physiotherapy colleagues for helping me in the formulation and practice of the hydrotherapy techniques.

Margaret Davies-Slate, Librarian, for title search and reference.

Anne Stewart, Secretary of Physiotherapy Department, for typing.

4

Karen Smith

HYDROTHERAPY IN NEUROLOGICAL REHABILITATION

INTRODUCTION

Hydrotherapy can be a very useful adjunct in the treatment of many neurological disorders taking its place in the overall rehabilitation programme of the patients. The main aims are threefold—therapeutic, recreational and psychological. A social component is involved in both the recreational and psychological aspects of these aims.

Hydrotherapy can be effective in reducing abnormal effects such as pain, altered muscle tone and the effect of gravity on weak movements allowing freer movement of the limbs and trunk, the re-education and strengthening of these movements by using the various properties of water on an immersed body. The re-education of righting and equilibrium reactions, body alignment and symmetry, breathing control and functional activities can also be facilitated.

Recreational water safety, swimming skills, socialization and the opportunity to participate in the other aquatic activities are provided. When movement is found to be easier as it is in water, then motivation occurs. This can lead to free and independent actions and the enhancement of confidence and self-esteem; thus psychological benefits accrue. However, it must be remembered that in certain conditions, such as stroke, there is loss of the body's ability to react to the effects of gravity and the environment in the normal way. The aim of much of the treatment for these patients is to achieve normal responses of the body to gravity, requiring the retraining to be performed in the normal environment. Hydrotherapy does have its place in the overall rehabilitation of these patients as movements or components of movement may be facilitated even though not entirely similar to such movements on land.

This chapter approaches the treatment of the neurological patient from the aspect of clinical signs and symptoms and these have been related to actual conditions. This is because, as physiotherapists in the neurological field an approach to treating each patient should be based on an initial full assessment to determine neurological signs and movement dysfunction (Carr and Shepherd, 1982). From these findings treatment aims are determined and the treatment programme should be developed according to these aims. On each occasion the patient is seen for treatment, the physiotherapist should reassess the patient's performance and revise the treatments accordingly. If this is true for land-based treatment programmes it is also true for hydrotherapy treatment programmes. Short-term goals for activity in water would be dependent on the land treatment aims, however, long-term goals would work towards total independence in water and swimming skills.

Indications for Hydrotherapy

Hydrotherapy for the neurological patient is indicated in any condition where there are alterations in muscle tone, loss of active range of movement due to weakness or paralysis, contractures which complicate the rehabilitation process and loss of balance, equilibrium reactions and coordination.

CLINICAL AIMS OF TREATMENT FOR NEUROLOGICAL DYSFUNCTION

Increased or Decreased Muscle Tone

Reference has been made to alterations in muscle tone which may occur in neurological conditions. There may have been an increase in muscle tone or a decrease in muscle tone or total loss of muscle tone.

Increased muscle tone, or hypertonia, can be of the spastic or rigid type (Atkinson, 1986). Both types are characterized by resistance to passive movement which in spasticity is velocity dependent and in rigidity the resistance is the same throughout the full range of passive movement whether moved slowly or quickly. Decreased muscle tone, or hypotonia, can be characterized by a reduced resistance to passive movement of the limb. Pool therapy is of value in all alterations of muscle tone; the warmth of the water temporarily decreases spasticity and together with the relaxation that takes place diminishes rigidity. Where muscle tone is decreased or lost voluntary movement is impaired or non-existent. The warmth of the water helps maintain the circulation with the concomitant effects of reducing trophic changes, joint mobility can be preserved and re-education of returning muscle power facilitated.

Specific techniques for altered muscle tone are indicated throughout this chapter. Such techniques should be carried out slowly and rhythmically. Swaying, swinging and rolling techniques form a valuable part of the treatment programme (Chapter 1).

Muscle Stretching

Prevention of contracture

In any condition where there is a loss of active range of movement due to weakness, increased muscle tone, inattention, dyspraxia or loss of sensation, the length of muscles and tendons as well as joint capsule mobility, must be maintained to prevent any shortening of these structures occurring which will prevent the full potential of any possible recovery being realized. Stretching is also necessary to maintain levels of function in the case of chronic conditions, such as multiple sclerosis. There is some debate about the necessity to passively stretch muscles to their full, particularly in the case of stroke patients, but this is not an appropriate arena in which to discuss the pros and cons of stretching. Scientific evidence shows that active movement is superior to passive movement in the maintenance of muscle length (Gossman *et al.*, 1982) and so active effort on the patient's part should be incorporated where possible, although if full range active movements were present, passive stretching would not be necessary. Stretching muscles through their full range is a basic but important part of the treatment of most neurologically damaged patients, not only for the purpose of preventing loss of range of movement of muscles, tendons and joint structures, but also in the reduction of increased muscle tone, and facilitation of antagonistic movement.

In some cases stretching can be a painful procedure, such as the hemiparetic patient where increased muscle tone can cause pain, or the Guillain Barré patient, where muscle tenderness is common and often severe. By performing these stretches in warm water pain can be significantly reduced. The warmth of the water may also bring relaxation of spasticity provided the water temperature is between 32–34°C. If the muscle tone is not increased and muscle tenderness is the problem, as in the Guillain Barré patient, the temperature may range between 34–37°C. Skinner and Thomson (1983) recommend a temperature range of 34–37°C but water temperatures above 34°C may cause the muscle tone to increase further, a view espoused by Margaret Rood (Stockmeyer, 1967). In the case of Guillain Barré syndrome, the warmth of the water reduces the muscle tenderness by inducing mild analgesia and relaxation of the muscles (Franchimont *et al.*, 1983).

Buoyancy also plays a part in relaxation, by the increased support of the body and limbs thereby reducing the effects of gravity which leads to reduction in tone and relaxation in response to changes in reflex activity (Franchimont *et al.*, 1983). Rhythmic repetitive movements performed slowly are also effective in reducing muscle tone, and in water these can be facilitated by the use of its buoyancy to reduce gravitational resistance to the movement, and in supporting the limb against gravity, thereby reducing the effort required to hold the limb in an antigravity position. This is an important factor because excess effort will cause associated reactions and increased tone.

EXAMPLES OF PROCEDURES

Hip adductor stretch

The hip adductor stretch of a Guillain Barré patient can be performed using an active-assisted movement, with full flotation of the patient, and incorporating rhythmical repetitive movements and momentum of the body.

Starting position: the patient should be floating in supine, fully supported by floats under the neck and pelvis and the feet where necessary.

Technique: the physiotherapist, with hands on the lateral surface of the thigh and ankle of the leg being stretched stands in water to a depth of approximately mid-thoracic level and instructs the patient to abduct the leg, giving only enough resistance to allow the movement to occur, and allowing the body of the patient to swing towards the physiotherapist in a circular motion. The end-of-range movement is assisted by changing the physiotherapist's hands to the medial surface of the leg and allowing the momentum of the patient's body to continue causing further hip abduction, before bringing the leg back to starting position, or completing the pattern by instructing the patient to abduct the leg. This is a modification of a Bad Ragaz technique, and the same method can be used to stretch many muscle groups where there is enough muscle power to initiate the momentum of the body.

Hemiplegic arm stretches

It should be noted that it is inadvisable to passively stretch the shoulder of a hemiplegic patient into any painful range of movement. This is because the scapula is commonly inhibited from normal movement by increased tone in the muscles of the shoulder girdle and the humero-scapular rhythm is disrupted. Unless the scapula moves freely on its own, or is manually moved by the physiotherapist in conjunction with humeral movement, the shoulder should not be forced into extremes of movement. To do so may cause pinching of the capsule or impingement of the humerus on the acromion process. Where relaxation of the shoulder girdle occurs in water, the scapula should move freely and this problem is less likely to occur. When the movement is active-assisted the scapular tone can be further inhibited by reciprocal inhibition, providing the effort required by the patient is not too great. The shoulder movements of flexion and extension can be performed in side lying on the unaffected side, supported on a plinth, with the water level to the top of the shoulder. Abduction and rotation of the shoulder can be performed with the patient in supine or sitting or standing upright, with the limb immersed to the top of the shoulder.

Patient's position: to stretch the elbow, forearm, wrist and fingers the *patient's position* is sitting or preferably lying in supine, with the water covering the limb to be stretched.

Technique: the physiotherapist, standing on the side of the patient and holding the arm to be stretched in abduction to 90°, faces in the direction of the patient's face. The arm is then fully extended at the elbow, using the physiotherapist's knee or the plinth as a pivot, and the forearm is fully supinated, the wrist, fingers and thumb extended while the thumb is held in abduction. The physiotherapist should have as little contact with the flexor surfaces as possible. This reflex inhibiting pattern (Bobath, 1978) should be held until the muscle tone can be felt to relax.

Hamstring stretches

Hamstring stretches can be either passive or active-assisted and depending on the ability of the patient to stand, can be performed in either standing or side lying.

Patient's position (side lying): the patient is side lying, supported on a plinth, with the water covering the uppermost hip.

Technique: it is necessary to have an assistant to hold the lower leg in the neutral position and fix the pelvis to prevent movement of the trunk. The upper leg is flexed at the hip by the physiotherapist, whose hands are placed behind the ankle and in front of the knee to maintain full knee extension, keeping the leg below the waterline. The fully extended hamstrings should be held in this position until the muscle tone relaxes, in the case of an upper motor neuron condition, and only momentarily for a lower motor neuron condition.

Patient's position (standing): the patient stands side on to the wall holding the bar with one hand and with the leg to be stretched outermost.

Technique: the physiotherapist, standing to the side and in front of the patient, asks the patient to lift the leg forward with knee straight. Using buoyancy to assist, the movement is continued, assisted also by the physiotherapist to attain a full range hamstring stretch, with the hands under the heel and over the knee preventing knee flexion. The other knee must be maintained in full extension.

REDUCING CONTRACTURES

Contractures should not occur with correct physiotherapy treatment but from time to time the physiotherapist is faced with trying to undo the damage which time and neglect so successfully create, making voluntary movement, washing and dressing so difficult for the patient or carer. The only way to reduce contractures, before resorting to serial plasters or surgery, is prolonged manual stretching and this can be very painful for the patient. For this reason immersion in warm water can help considerably by relieving some of the pain, promoting relaxation and improving the blood supply to the affected muscles (Franchimont *et al.*, 1983). The techniques for stretching out contractures are the same as those used for their prevention, with the added need to prolong the stretch for as long as can be tolerated by the patient and to repeat the stretches many times, gradually increasing the pressure on the muscle groups, and working within the patient's tolerance. The best rule is not to allow the contractures to occur in the first place!

Muscle Strengthening

Conditions requiring strengthening exercises include; Guillain Barré syndrome, peripheral neuropathies, multiple sclerosis, Parkinson's disease, Friedreich's ataxia, myelopathies and muscular dystrophies, motor neuron diseases, multisystems degeneration, transverse myelitis, polymyositis and late stage strokes.

Much of the hydrotherapy for neurological conditions can be said to aim towards the strengthening of weak muscles in the case of lower motor neuron disorders and muscular dystrophies, and the strengthening of a movement or improving a movement pattern in the case of the stroke patient where muscle strength is not the major problem. Information is available on the mechanisms of the effect of water on an immersed body and the hydrodynamic principles (Skinner and Thomson, 1983) all of which can be utilized at various stages in the patient's progress so these will not be repeated here.

The process of strengthening muscles is straightforward and examples of exercises for this purpose can be found in other chapters of this book. But where increased muscle tone is involved the resistance given to the body part must not be enough to cause associated reactions or increased muscle tone in that or any other part of the body. This must be carefully monitored by the physiotherapist and the patient must be taught to be aware of this and not exert excessive force when attempting a movement.

Associated reactions may also be increased where inadequate support is given, where handling is of poor quality, where there is lack of stability and where anxiety is present. The importance of adequate support and good handling is, therefore, emphasized. Obtaining and maintaining stability and overcoming anxiety can be brought about by teaching mental adjustment and balance restoration (see p. 17). The assumption of stable shapes, such as a 'sitting' posture with the legs apart and right angles at hips, knees and ankles with the arms forward enhances stability and this can be further increased if the head and arms are used to assist the maintenance of this position against any disturbing influences, for instance, turbulence (Reid Campion, 1985).

RE-EDUCATION OF MOTOR PATTERNS

Where increased tone is present movement patterns will be abnormal. It follows therefore, that to normalize the patterns of movement the muscle tone must first be normalized by the use of prolonged stretching through positioning of the patient, buoyancy and the warmth of the water. Once the muscle tone is reduced, the movement patterns may be re-educated, by working the patient's muscle groups in those or individual movements, outside the synergic or abnormal movement patterns. Care must be taken by the physiotherapist to avoid causing the muscle tone to increase during exercise. The use of resistance in any form must be avoided for those muscle groups with moderate to severe increased muscle tone, as its use will only exacerbate the problem further by increasing the tone in these muscles and inhibiting movement of the antagonists. Hydrotherapy can be usefully employed in the treatment of such patients by utilizing the assistive effects of buoyancy on a limb, thereby reducing gravitational resistance and excessive effort on the patient's part. As already indicated immersion in warm water helps to reduce muscle tone and this state may last for a short period afterwards. An appropriate time to carry out the land-based programme might well be during this period of decreased muscle tone.

Re-education of motor patterns may involve the head, trunk and upper and lower limbs as a whole unit or broken down into similar components. The major patterns of standing to sitting to lying, and from lying to sitting, sitting to standing, turning and rolling in the horizontal can be facilitated. Such actions form vertical and lateral rotation in the water and are used to teach mental adjustment and balance restoration (Chapter 1).

EXAMPLES OF PROCEDURES

Standing to lying to standing through sitting

Patient's position: the patient stands with the water at xiphisternum level.

Technique: the physiotherapist stands behind the patient and places the heels of the hands in the patient's waist with the fingers pointing down over the patient's buttocks. The patient is instructed to 'sit', that is, to bend the knees and hips and to get the shoulders under the water and lift the arms forwards so that they are held just below the surface. The feet should be placed about hip width apart. The head is then taken backwards so that it is placed on the physiotherapist's shoulder. The lower limbs rise towards the surface and they are slowly extended.

From the lying position the patient is required to bend the knees towards the chest, to bring the head and hands forwards, to rotate the body forwards to the upright position and then to lower the feet and stabilize the body in the 'sitting' position again with the arms forwards prior to standing erect. Precise balance is required in sitting and standing, especially of the head on the spine, against the turbulence created by the forward movement. Total flexion and extension of the head, trunk and lower limbs is achieved, the arms reach symmetrically or asymmetrically as required. Initially in some instances the hands may need to be linked to achieve a degree of symmetry but the aim should be towards the forward action being created with symmetry and the hands being unclasped. This exercise is readily broken down into small tasks; for example standing to sitting; arms forwards; from sitting to lying and so on.

Turning in the vertical

Patient's position: the patient stands in front of the physiotherapist facing away with the arms forwards.

Technique: if the patient is turning to the right the head is turned in that direction and the left arm and leg are taken across the midline to produce the turning action which continues with the feet taking small steps until the patient is facing forwards again. The physiotherapist can facilitate the turning action by 'patting' the patient around with the hands at the waist. This turning can be achieved by the head, by the arm being taken across the body and by the crossing of the leg, but the head is the critical component.

Rolling in the horizontal

Patient's position: the patient lies supine supported under the trunk at a right angle to one side of the physiotherapist who supports the patient at the level of the inferior angle of the scapulae with the arm on that side.

Technique: to create a roll through 360° in front of the physiotherapist the patient turns the head towards the physiotherapist and brings the outer arm and leg across the body. As the patient's outer arm is brought across the body the physiotherapist's free arm supports and guides it as it moves, without coming into contact with the patient's thorax. With the rolling action complete, the patient will be at a right angle to the physiotherapist, supported as already described but on the opposite side of the physiotherapist to which the rolling movement commenced. This rolling action may be carried out in flexion, when both knees would be brought towards the chest, or in a more extended position where the outer leg is brought across the other leg at the knee or ankle.

As a progression, horizontal rolling can be carried out by the physiotherapist giving less support. The physiotherapist stands facing the patient, the hands at the patient's waist. A step is taken to one side and the patient assumes the supine lying position. The physiotherapist needs to stabilize the body position so places the leg nearest to the patient directly below the centre of balance of the patient's body and bends the knee keeping the foot flat on the floor of the pool. The outer leg is abducted and extended. The physiotherapist is now in a lunge position. The only other action the physiotherapist needs to take is to 'pat' the patient's body around with the hands remaining at waist level.

For the safety of the patient and the physiotherapist all rolling actions should take place towards the physiotherapist. Since it is advisable that the patient be able to roll in both directions the physiotherapist must move around the patient's head whilst supporting the body under its centre of balance (Reid Campion, 1985).

RE-EDUCATION OF BALANCE AND EQUILIBRIUM REACTIONS

Conditions suitable for balance retraining include: Parkinson's disease, supra-nuclear palsy, cerebellar and multisystems degeneration, multiple sclerosis, transverse myelitis, hypoxic encephalopathy, brainstem CVA, cerebellar CVA, later stage hemiparetic rehabilitation, Guillain Barré syndrome and polyneuropathies.

The re-education of the equilibrium reactions in the hemiparetic patient is best done on land in the early stages of rehabilitation. This is because the aim is to retrain the body to react normally to the effects of gravity and loss of equilibrium. In the water the patient's reactions will be different to those on land, due to the added properties the water possesses.

Hydrotherapy, however, does have a place in balance re-training in those conditions mentioned above. It is largely the head and to a lesser degree the trunk which initiate movement in the water, thus head and trunk control are of extreme importance in the re-education of balance and functional activities. ' "Where the head goes the body follows", if this is true on land it is equally true in water where the head controls the position of the body and feet entirely' (Reid Campion, 1985, p. 9). Balance retraining should be introduced at later stages in the rehabilitation of the hemiparetic patient, once the correct responses have been gained on land. Here, use can be made of the supporting effect of the buoyancy of the water to gain the patient's confidence and reduce the fear of falling. Turbulence may also be used to threaten balance, (see following example) in order to elicit the correct response from the patient i.e. the righting, tilting and propping reactions which the hemiparetic patient must have first learnt on land. These can be further strengthened in water with added confidence to the patient that he will not fall and be hurt. A further use of these properties of water is to re-accustom the patient to water following the onset of the stroke or other neurological conditions, if swimming is a normal activity for recreation.

EXAMPLES OF PROCEDURES

Sitting balance exercises

Patient's position: the patient 'sits' in the water with the shoulders under the water, the arms forward and the hips, knees and ankles flexed as near to a right angle as possible with the legs about hip width apart.

Technique: the physiotherapist stands behind the patient stabilizing the patient at the waist until a stable position is established. The physiotherapist, gently at first, creates turbulence behind the patient's back. Using the head, shoulders, arms and hands the patient endeavours to maintain a stable sitting position. The physiotherapist gauges the amount of turbulence to be applied at any moment, also where it is to be placed will be determined by the patient's problem. Increasing turbulence demands more balance and coordination as it threatens the patient's stability. Placing turbulence in varying directions progressing to walking around the patient and reversing the direction makes greater demands still on the patient's ability to control the body position.

Patient's position: the patient sits on a stool with the water level to shoulder level.

Technique: the physiotherapist should either 'sit' or kneel in front of the patient to give confidence against falling when beginning the exercise. Later as the patient becomes more confident the physiotherapist may assume a position behind the patient. The physiotherapist tilts the stool sideways, forwards and backwards and encourages the patient to react correctly by using his head and trunk to prevent loss of balance. To progress the exercise the physiotherapist can create turbulence in the water around the patient again threatening his balance in all directions and encouraging the appropriate reactions in the head, trunk and limbs.

Standing balance exercises

Patient's position: the patient stands away from the sides of the pool in water deep enough to reach the xiphisternum level. The legs should be apart sideways giving a wider base and thus more stability laterally.

Technique: the physiotherapist should stand in front of the patient and may progress to standing behind the patient as confidence improves. The physiotherapist then creates turbulence around the patient as previously described in the first sitting balance exercise. Static balance against the created turbulence is demanded of the patient and again greater balance and coordination is necessary as the amount and degree of turbulence is applied in various places and directions. This exercise can be further progressed by reducing the standing base by the patient bringing the feet closer together.

Patient's position: the patient stands as in the above exercise with a wide base at first.

Technique: the physiotherapist stands in front of the patient initially progressing to standing behind the patient as confidence improves. The physiotherapist then threatens the patient's balance by displacing the pelvis manually in various directions, tilting the patient slowly at first, and increasing in speed as the patient's reactions improve. The shoulders may also be used to displace the body and produce balance and equilibrium reactions.

The use of a narrower base and increasing the speed and size of the displacement will demand greater reactions from the patient. Turbulence will be created as the patient's body is displaced, the reactions will take place against that force, and the responses became faster and more complete.

Further progressions of both the sitting and standing balance exercises can be obtained in the following manner.

Sitting or standing balance exercise

Patient's position: the patient is 'sitting' as previously described immersed in the water so that the shoulders are just under the surface and away from the sides of the pool. Alternatively, the patient stands with the feet apart sideways immersed in the water so that the shoulders are covered.

Technique: these exercises are for the patient who is able to balance independently; the physiotherapist standing close enough to the patient as safety allows. The patient creates his own turbulence in the water around him, as well as pushing himself off balance using water resistance or impedance in the following ways:

● Firstly, using the arms, the patient makes a fast swinging movement, bringing them forwards from the body to the water surface and keeping the elbows and fingers extended, then bringing them downward towards his sides and continuing the movement backwards behind him, returning them to his sides and repeating the movement.
● Secondly, the patient can make a rotational movement of the trunk, starting with his arms abducted to just below the water's surface with the elbows and fingers extended. He then swings one arm forwards and the other arm backwards, keeping the arms just below the surface, and rotating the upper trunk at the same time. The movement is then reversed, rotating the trunk and arms in the opposite direction.

These manoeuvres make upright posture and balance more difficult to maintain, and the trunk and legs must work hard to correct the balance. Progression of the exercises can be made by increasing the speed of the movements to create more turbulence, using batons held in the hands to increase the water resistance or impedance, and turbulence, and also by standing on one leg. Further methods of improving balance and confidence in the water in neurologically disabled patients can be found using the Halliwick method of teaching swimming, floating and moving in water (Martin, 1981; Reid Campion, 1985).

GAIT RE-TRAINING (see also p 28)

This sub-section is divided into two parts. The first looks at the re-education of gait in lower motor neuron conditions and spinal cord conditions. The second considers upper motor neuron lesions involving the cerebral hemispheres, cerebellum and brainstem.

Lower Motor Neuron and Spinal Cord Lesions

The group of conditions which fall into these categories includes Guillain Barré syndrome, peripheral neuropathies, polymyositis, polyneuropathy, multiple sclerosis, transverse myelitis and peripheral nerve lesions. This group may also include the muscular dystrophies and myelopathies, some brainstem and cerebellar CVA's as well as anoxic encephalopathies. NB *Conditions involving the spinal cord (such as multiple sclerosis) are dealt with here, as they generally have many additional problems associated with the condition, and are not the same as a traumatic spinal lesion.*

These types of patients will gain the most benefit from gait re-education work in the water as their problems arise from weakness of muscle contraction and in some conditions increased tone as opposed to the problems arising from cortical lesions which involve loss of normal motor patterns. The water's buoyancy gives support to the very weak patient, allowing him to stand and walk much earlier than would be possible on land, even with the use of splinting and walking aids, and greatly reduces the possibility of joint damage caused by early weight bearing on unprotected joints due to severe muscle weakness or lack of proprioception. From a psychological viewpoint, this can be a great boost to the morale of a patient suffering from a long illness which has confined him to a bed or wheelchair, or to the person who has a chronic condition and is now unable to walk on land. Early walking training in the pool will also benefit the patient by stimulating the postural reactions of the trunk, and the upright posture and water pressure will benefit bladder function and the circulation of the lower limbs. Gait retraining on land, as a progression from the pool, will be facilitated by the patient having initially learnt the walking patterns in water and gained the necessary trunk control in the upright position.

Patient's position: in very severe cases, the patient may need to start walking practice in the kneeling position, but the majority can start in standing. The water level necessary will depend on the patient's ability and muscle strength; the weakest patients will need the water to reach the shoulders, giving the maximum support.

Method: there are many ways to give the patient support for walking in the pool and the method chosen by the physiotherapist will depend on the disability of the patient and most importantly on safety considerations (i.e. whether or not the patient is able to float or swim independently). The following are different ways to give the patient support while walking in the pool; the patient holds the wall bar, parallel bars, the patient walks holding a float in front of him; the physiotherapist stands facing the patient and uses a forearm grip with both hands, the physiotherapist stands behind the patient holding the shoulders or pelvis, the patient uses a weighted walking frame.

In addition to progression from more support to less support, the activity can be progressed by walking in shallower water which will give the patient less support, increasing the effects of gravity on the body, and by asking the patient to walk faster, the resistance against his movements will be increased, giving heavier work to the muscles.

Upper Motor Neuron Lesions

This group of patients constitutes those with strokes affecting the cerebral cortex and pyramidal pathways as well as other conditions such as multiple sclerosis and bacterial encephalopathies causing lesions in these areas of the brain.

These patients, who have a central disruption to their patterns of movement giving rise to abnormal synergies or patterns of increased muscle tone and abnormal responses to gravitational forces, will in general benefit from gait re-education in a normal environment.

They need to experience the normal feedback on land in order to relearn the normal responses necessary for upright posture and balance. It is postulated that the upright posture may be facilitated in water if the appropriate depth is used.

Balance is readily re-educated in water because the difficulty in obtaining stability in this medium makes considerable demands on balance and coordination. Constant correction of the gait pattern is essential with these patients if the desired normal or near normal pattern of walking is to be achieved. It is not always easy to see and correct faults in water, nevertheless weight shifting laterally and forwards and backwards, as preliminaries to walking with the dangers of falling diminished due to the support of the water can be beneficial. Some parts of the gait sequence do benefit from practice in the pool where buoyancy and the relaxation effects may facilitate the movement for example and inhibit abnormal movement patterns. Flexion of the leg in the swing phase is facilitated by buoyancy. Exercises to develop knee flexion and knee extension are useful (p. 90). Other means of re-educating gait which are most effective in improving balance and coordination along with increasing range of movement in all the movements of the joints involved and the strengthening of muscle groups are described in Chapter 1 (p. 21).

BREATHING EXERCISES

Breathing exercises to improve thoracic expansion and breath control performed in the water, have a useful place in the treatment of many neurological conditions, in which these functions are impaired.

Conditions which may benefit from these exercises may include stroke, particularly bilateral CVA's and brainstem CVA's bulbar involvement, Parkinson's disease, Friedreich's ataxia, Guillain Barré syndrome and other chronic degenerative conditions affecting the thoracic muscles, such as multiple sclerosis.

Exercises for Thoracic Expansion Laterally

The principle applied here is the prolonged stretch to facilitate relaxation of the muscles of the rib cage, and a quick stretch to facilitate expansion, followed by resistance to the movement, giving the patient increased awareness of the chest expansion in the targeted area (Skinner and Thomson, 1983).

Patient's position: the patient is supported on a plinth, in supine lying submerged in water to the level of the neck, with both legs held to one side by the physiotherapist.

Technique: the physiotherapist stands to the side of the patient with one hand on the lateral aspect of the thigh near the knee and the other hand on the lateral aspect of the rib cage. Just before inspiration, the legs are pushed further sideways away from the side to be expanded, giving a stretch to the muscles of the thorax, while with the other hand a quick stretch is applied to the intercostals and accessory muscles by a quick press and release downwards and inwards. The physiotherapist's hand maintains some pressure on the ribs as the patient breathes in, and is asked to push his ribs against the hand pressure simultaneously. The breath should be held momentarily, and then gently expired, as the physiotherapist releases pressure on the chest and legs. The exercise should be timed to correspond with the patient's breathing pattern, and performed several times. It is then important to rest the patient before continuing, to prevent the patient hyperventilating.

Exercises can be done during the rest periods. This technique can be applied to encourage expansion of different parts of the thoracic cage, by exerting the stretch on the appropriate part by moving the legs and lower trunk away from that aspect, and applying the quick stretch and resistance over the thoracic area targeted.

Exercises for Breath Control

There are many exercises designed to improve breath control in water for swimming or floating activities for children, which can be found in *Hydrotherapy in Paediatrics* by Reid Campion, 1985. Many of these are suitable for use with adults, to improve the control of expiration for voice control, in those patients where poor coordination affects speech. Often it may be valuable to work on this problem in conjunction with a speech therapist, and more information can be found in Chapter 3.

FITNESS AND PSYCHOLOGICAL EFFECTS

It is relevant here to stress the importance of fitness for those patients with chronic neurological disease or dysfunction. In many cases, swimming or exercise in water is the only activity in which they are able to participate in which their level of fitness may be improved or maintained, or where they can derive enjoyment from a medium, giving them relative freedom to move about independently of a wheelchair and/or walking aid. For those patients who have suffered a disability with a sudden onset, such as stroke, water is a medium to which they can return for recreation as well as to improve fitness levels. The achieving of confidence in water is often a patient's first step back into leading a normal if changed lifestyle. The Halliwick method (Martin, 1981; Skinner and Thomson, 1983) can be used to introduce the disabled person to using the medium of water for swimming and enjoyment of new freedom.

Conditions

This section has been included to allow for descriptions of the treatment of several conditions which include features not common to most other neurological conditions and thus require special mention with regard to their treatment in water.

Stroke

In rehabilitating the hemiparetic patient, the aims of treatment include normalizing muscle tone, normalizing movement patterns and re-educating the reactions of the body to gravity and other forces. Fundamental to all of these aims is the normalizing of tone in the trunk and limbs. Until tone becomes normal, movement cannot become normal and therefore, any physiotherapy programme, on land or in the water, must make this the single most important consideration when assessing the effects of any movement the patient is asked to make or assume.

When commencing hydrotherapy treatment the first thing which must be assessed is the effect of the patient's immersion in water. Sometimes the patient's fear of water will cause an increase in tone. This may be overcome by an explanation to the patient of the characteristics and properties of water, by indicating any possible rotational effects that can occur due to the patient's altered shape and density and informing the patient as to the action he should take to counteract any rotation. Once in the water mental adjustment and balance restoration can be developed practically (p. 17). Occasionally the heat may cause an increase in muscle tone (Stockmeyer, 1967) although there are no physiological studies to support this phenomenon. Often this effect will decrease with continued immersion, but the physiotherapist should be aware of the possibility of its ocurrence and if improvement does not take place during several sessions, hydrotherapy should be discontinued. If these problems are overcome or do not arise, water is an excellent medium for promoting general relaxation, which in turn will facilitate relaxation of specific muscle groups. The following are some examples of methods to reduce increased muscle tone in the stroke patient.

Reducing tone in the trunk

Bobath techniques focus on decreasing or normalizing the tone in the trunk, especially of the muscles in the lumbar region, the pelvic girdle and shoulder girdle, key areas of tone control which will influence the tone in the peripheries. Some of these techniques can be adapted for use in the hydrotherapy pool.

Patient's position: flotation of the patient, fully supported by floats under the neck, pelvis and each foot, is an excellent position in which to manipulate the trunk in the water.

Technique: the physiotherapist stands between the patient's legs, holding the thighs or iliac crests firmly within both hands. Once the patient is confident and relaxed in this position the physiotherapist tells the patient to further 'let go' or 'relax'. Then rhythmically and slowly the physiotherapist moves the lower half of the body from side to side, swinging in a wide arc, allowing the turbulence of the water to move the upper half of the body in the opposite direction. This will gently stretch the lower trunk muscles, and as they relax, the pelvis can be rotated slightly on each swing, further releasing tone in the pelvic girdle muscles.

Reducing tone in the shoulder girdle

Patient's position: this exercise can be performed either with the patient seated and submerged to just above the shoulder level, or in side lying on the unaffected side on a plinth, again making sure the uppermost shoulder is submerged.

Technique:the physiotherapist stands facing the patient, and supports the patient's affected arm in shoulder flexion to 90°, making sure the elbow is extended. Alternatively the arm may be supported by floats. An inflatable arm splint of the type used by Margaret Johnstone (Johnstone, 1982) is a particularly useful piece of equipment for this purpose as it provides not only flotation for the arm, but holds the arm in the reflex inhibiting position of elbow extension, supination, wrist and finger extension and abduction of the thumb.

This leaves the physiotherapist's hands free to provide greater control of the patient's movements. The physiotherapist passively moves the scapula into protraction and rotation laterally, relaxing the shoulder girdle muscles using rhythmic repetitive movements. As the muscles become more relaxed the physiotherapist asks the patient to gently protract the scapula with assistance, progressing to independent movement provided no increase in tone occurs in the scapular and shoulder muscle groups.

This exercise prepares the patient for further active work on the shoulder, elbow and hand by producing a decrease in general arm tone. (Further methods of reducing tone are described in Chapter 1, p. 28, and in this chapter, p. 71.) The effect of reducing tone in the trunk and proximal muscle groups is a flow over to the muscles of the peripheries, in preparation for active movement retraining in other more distal muscle groups.

Retraining Movement

The retraining of movement should follow directly on from the initial relaxation and tone reducing manoeuvres described above and in fact should be combined for effective results, the physiotherapist constantly assessing any tonal change during an exercise. Should tone become increased due to excessive exertion or incorrect movements, the physiotherapist should repeat the manoeuvres described above and reduce the tone again before continuing with the activity. The aim in the treatment of stroke patients should be to teach normal patterns of movement and to inhibit abnormal patterns or synergies (Brunnstrom, 1970).

Hydrotherapy can be effective in the re-education of both upper and lower limb movement patterns, not only because of its relaxation effects, but also by using buoyancy to minimize the effect of gravity on the limbs, thereby reducing excessive effort on the patient's behalf and minimizing the occurrence of associated reactions and increases in tone. For example, when trying to progress a patient's arm movement patterns of elbow extension on land, from being able to perform active elbow extension in supine with the shoulder flexed to 90°, the next aim would be to attempt the elbow extension with the patient in sitting and the shoulder flexed to 90°. The effort required for the patient to maintain his shoulder in flexion in sitting will cause an increase in tone in the arm flexors and inhibit the extension movements in the elbow, wrist and fingers. In water, using buoyancy to support the arm in shoulder flexion, the extension patterns may be facilitated, and can be practised as an interim step until the patient is able to produce the movement out of the water. These same principles can be applied to many limb movements, working outside the synergies and providing an interim step when moving from one position of a limb or body to a more advanced position.

EXAMPLES OF PROCEDURES

Knee flexion in standing

Knee flexion with the hip in a neutral or extended position, is often a difficult movement to obtain in the hemiparetic patient, but necessary if a normal or near normal gait pattern is to be achieved. The process of re-learning the movement may start in side lying, progressing to prone lying; however, to progress from prone to standing is difficult and may benefit from an interim step in the water.

Patient's position: the patient stands facing the pool wall, holding the bar for balance. The hips should remain in the neutral position throughout the exercise, and no hip flexion must be allowed.

Technique: the patient is asked to slowly attempt knee flexion of the affected leg, while not allowing the hip to flex or pelvic retraction to occur. The movement is assisted by the buoyancy of the water, and the physiotherapist must be careful not to allow any increase in tone, especially in the muscles around the lower trunk and pelvis. Progression can be made, once the patient can achieve this movement well, to extending the affected hip while maintaining the knee at 90° flexion. From there the movement can be incorporated into the gait pattern by breaking this down into its component parts, practising each part separately and eventually putting them together into a whole pattern.

Horizontal shoulder abduction

Horizontal abduction of the shoulder is often a difficult movement for the hemiparetic patient to achieve out of the water, as shoulder abduction forms part of the flexor synergy and predisposes the arm to increasing tone in the elbow and forearm flexors. By doing the exercise in water, the use of buoyancy, again, diminishes the effort required to support the arm against gravity and helps to reduce or eliminate the increase in flexor tone at the elbow and hand.

Patient's position: the patient may be sitting or standing, the water level just covering the shoulders.

Technique: the patient's affected arm may be supported on floats, an inflatable splint, or by the physiotherapist if the patient does not have the necessary control to maintain the arm in the starting position of 90° flexion at the shoulder. The inflatable splint is necessary only if the patient cannot maintain the elbow in extension. From this position the patient is asked to move his arm slowly across the surface of the water into full abduction, while being careful not to allow any flexion at the elbow. The arm is slowly returned to the starting position by the patient and the movement is repeated. As the patient's shoulder control progresses, progression of the exercise is obtained by increasing the speed of movement, but always within the limits set by any increase in flexor tone.

IMPORTANT POINTS TO NOTE

When treating the hemiparetic patient, it should be stressed that all movements should be performed with resistance minimized in order to avoid any increase in tone in the body part being exercised or in other parts of the body. To this end, certain rules can be applied to the treatment of those patients where this is likely to occur:

● the patient should always make slow movements to reduce the effect of water resistance and turbulence

- the patient should not be asked to make a movement using a float and buoyancy as resistance
- the use of batons to increase surface area and hence resistance should not be attempted
- the physiotherapist should always be observant for signs of increased tone and modify the treatment accordingly
- the use of additional turbulence by the physiotherapist with some patients with poor balance may cause a general increase in tone.

The Painful Hemiplegic Shoulder

The painful hemiplegic shoulder is a problem which occurs regularly and sparks a great deal of debate regarding the cause and treatment of the condition. In fact the painful hemiplegic shoulder can be described as two separate conditions.

The shoulder-hand syndrome

This is an autonomic dystrophy, involving not only the shoulder but also the periphery of the upper limb. The causes of this condition are not known, although many theories have been put forward (Caillet, 1980).

Capsulitis or tendonitis

This is a common cause of shoulder pain, which is generally caused by incorrect handling or positioning of the shoulder, or by overuse and incorrect exercise techniques.

These two conditions are dealt with separately in relation to their causes and treatment, although many of the techniques of treatment and individual exercises are beneficial to both conditions for slightly different reasons.

THE SHOULDER-HAND SYNDROME

This syndrome is characterized by pain in the shoulder, usually elicited by the movement of flexion abduction and lateral rotation in a painful arc of varying degree according to the severity of the condition. In severe cases, the pain can be elicited by any movement or merely by the weight of the arm hanging dependent. In addition oedema of the hand and wrist is present, which in turn gives rise to pain on movement of the affected joints, especially in the fingers where the increase of pressure due to oedema in the compartments of the tendon sheaths causes a splinting effect. The condition is self limiting and will eventually recover, but if the arm is left untreated until this occurs, the patient will be left with a clawed and ankylosed hand and a frozen shoulder. The preventative treatment is simply to reduce the oedema and maintain the mobility of the involved joints and the muscle and tendon lengths, by joint mobilization and stretching.

In the early stages of the condition, the oedema will usually respond best to the use of ice, combined with elevation and massage if necessary. This can be either manual or using an intermittent pressure machine. The application of a fitted lycra glove after treatment, to be worn during the day, will help maintain the effects of the treatment for longer periods. However, in the more chronic stage of the condition, the use of warmth in treating the oedema may be more effective and here hydrotherapy can be used to reduce oedema, improve blood circulation, and aid with relaxation of increased tone around the shoulder and scapula. Having achieved these effects, mobilization of the scapula, shoulder, wrist and finger joints can be performed while the joints are immersed in the water, using the techniques of Maitland (Maitland, 1977) or Kaltenborn (Kaltenborn, 1980) for peripheral joint mobilization. Following mobilization, the muscles of the elbow, forearm, wrist and finger muscles should be slowly, passively stretched as fully as the patient can tolerate. The shoulder movements, should be active or active-assisted movements, which can often be effectively and less painfully performed using buoyancy to assist the movement, as described on p. 94. Movement of the shoulder should at all times be within a painfree range of movement, and scapula movements can be assisted manually by the physiotherapist during the exercises.

CAPSULITIS AND TENDONITIS OF THE SHOULDER

The causes of pain in the hemiplegic shoulder due to capsulitis or tendonitis are as follows; incorrect handling of the shoulder by staff or by the patient, poor positioning of the shoulder, incorrect exercise techniques and excessive repetitive exercises. The prevention of this condition can be effected through education of hospital staff, the patient and family as to the correct handling and positioning of the arm and shoulder, and patients with inattention of the affected side or sensory problems may benefit from extra protection in the form of a shoulder support. Physiotherapy treatment of the shoulder movements must be carefully supervised to prevent incorrect movements being performed, or overuse of the shoulder by excessive repetitive movements. All shoulder movements must be within a painfree range of movements, and this is commonly aided by mobilization and assisted movement of the scapula by the physiotherapist. If the condition develops, this treatment is very effective if performed in water, using the warmth to reduce pain and aid relaxation of muscle spasm and increased tone in the muscles of the shoulder girdle. Exercises for the shoulder can be performed in the same manner as for shoulder-hand syndrome, using buoyancy to assist the movement and working within the limits of pain.

EXAMPLES OF PROCEDURES

Shoulder abduction

Patient's position: the patient may be sitting or standing ensuring that the water level is above the shoulders.

Technique: the patient actively abducts the arm slowly assisted by the water's buoyancy, and if necessary the physiotherapist should assist the rotation of the scapula. To gain further range of movement, the patient can incline his body in the direction of the affected arm, while holding a wall bar, with the other hand to support the body at the desired angle.

Shoulder flexion

Patient's position: the same position as the exercise above.

Technique: the patient slowly flexes the shoulder, again assisted by buoyancy. The same principle can be applied to increase the range of movement gently, by moving the body forward towards the direction of movement, whilst holding a bar with the other hand.

Horizontal abduction-adduction

This exercise is described in the section on the stroke patient. Note, however that in all these exercises the scapula movement should be closely observed by the physiotherapist to ensure correct movement in sequence with the humerus, and if necessary manually assisted.

Mobilization Techniques

Mobilization of the affected joints is most important where there is loss of range of joint movement due to pain or oedema, in order to prevent structural shortening of ligaments and joint capsules and adhesion formation. The techniques of Maitland and Kaltenborn can be effectively performed in the water with good results, aided by the pain relieving and relaxing properties of the warm water. The techniques need not be modified for use in water, although the patient or limb may require more stabilizing.

ATAXIA

There are two types of ataxia, cerebellar ataxia and sensory ataxia.

Cerebellar ataxia—is caused by lesions in the cerebellum, or spino-cerebellar pathways and is characterized by intention tremor, incoordination, dysdiadochokinesias and dysmetria. Conditions which may lead to cerebellar ataxia are; multiple sclerosis, cerebellar degeneration, brainstem CVA, cerebellar CVA and Friedreich's ataxia. Whilst some patients with cerebellar ataxia may not respond well to hydrotherapy aimed at improving the balance, in the author's experience, strengthening of the muscles, particularly the proximal groups of the trunk, shoulder girdle and pelvic girdle, does play a part in improving the control of movement. The use of both the isotonic and isometric patterns of the Bad Ragaz techniques can be effectively applied to patients with cerebellar ataxia. Additionally hydrodynamic exercises as described in Chapter 2 have proved useful in the treatment of this condition.

Sensory ataxia—is due to the de-afferentiation of a limb or limbs causing loss of sensory feedback. The proprioceptive pathways are the most important factor in this type of ataxia, making visual feedback to the patient very important for control of the affected part. Conditions causing this form of ataxia include syringomyelia, peripheral neuropathies, Guillain Barré syndrome, peripheral nerve lesions, stroke, Friedreich's ataxia and multiple sclerosis.

Walking in the water is difficult for these patients due to the difficulty of vision below the water line, as this is necessary to compensate for the loss of sensory feedback. Many of these patients also complain of a disorientation effect in water. For these patients, hydrotherapy may not be indicated; however, in the author's experience, much benefit can be gained in the areas of strength, endurance and psychological well-being using swimming, and Bad Ragaz techniques, for those patients who are able to tolerate this medium.

PARKINSON'S DISEASE

Parkinson's disease is dealt with separately because the condition has many features which are not common to other conditions. Two exceptions are Supranuclear palsy and some forms of multisystems degeneration which may have some features in common with Parkinson's disease. The features are namely bradykinesia, rigidity, especially in the trunk, paucity of movement, weakness of extensor groups of limb and trunk muscles, reduced thoracic expansion and loss of postural and equilibrium responses. Hydrotherapy in these conditions can be effective as the water often has the effect of reducing rigidity and the 'heaviness' of the body and facilitating freer movement, allowing a fuller range of movements of the trunk and limbs to be achieved. Thus these patients are able to improve extensor strength of the trunk and limbs, reduce or prevent tightness and contracture of the flexor groups of muscles, improve the reciprocal and rotational movements, maintain improved posture and improve the equilibrium responses. Akinesia and bradykinesia is often lessened in water, possibly due to the abnormal stimulus of the water pressure and turbulence on the body giving an increased sensory feedback to the brain. The resistance the water gives to movement may also play a part in facilitating the initiation of movement, just as the use of a goal or an obstacle to a movement may be employed by a patient to overcome the akinesia which is so frustrating for these patients. In some cases, the warmth of the water does not produce the desired response of relaxation of the rigidity and may even cause an increase in symptoms. In these cases hydrotherapy treatment is not indicated. (Skinner and Thomson, 1983). Cooler water may prove beneficial.

EXAMPLES OF PROCEDURES

Trunk rotation exercise

Patient's position: the patient stands with feet wide apart to prevent loss of balance and to fix the lower half of the body firmly. Alternatively, the patient may sit on a stool. The water level should be just above the shoulders.

Technique: the patient starts with the arms stretched straight out to the sides just below the surface of the water, and rotates the upper trunk using the arms to initiate the movement, by swinging one arm forward, the other backward along the water surface. The movement should be slow and rhythmical, gradually increasing in speed, but ensuring that the full range of trunk rotation is achieved. Increasing the speed causes an increase in resistance and turbulence, and this may be further increased by holding batons in the hands. This exercise will also help improve the patient's balance as the water resistance and turbulence produced make the patient's trunk and leg muscles work hard to counteract these forces and maintain the upright posture.

Strengthening extensor groups of legs and trunk

Patient's position: the patient is supported in full supine flotation, with floats under the neck and pelvis.

Technique: The Bad Ragaz techniques of trunk extension with rotation and reciprocally trunk flexion with rotation are effective ways of working on trunk flexors and extensors. This is a modification of the propioceptive neuromuscular facilitation (PNF) pattern used on land. The physiotherapist stands at the patient's feet, the water depth to approximately the mid-thoracic level, with a stable stance, preferably with her back to the wall and hands holding the patient's ankles. The patient is asked to flex the hips, knees and trunk to one side. By resisting this movement, the patient is caused to move towards the physiotherapist. At the end of range of flexion the patient pushes away from the physiotherapist by extending the legs and trunk and then rotating in the opposite direction. The resistance to the movement can be varied by altering the speed of the movement—the greater the speed, the more resistance is produced.

An alternate method of working the flexor and extensor groups of the trunk and legs, requires a set of parallel bars situated at water level in water deep enough to allow the patient to fully extend the trunk and legs without touching the bottom of the pool, while facing the bars with both arms stretched over the nearest bar and gripping the bar farthest away from him.

Technique: the patient, using a grip over the bars as a pivot point, starts the exercise with both legs extended behind and floating prone on the surface of the water. The legs, with the knees straight and the feet together, are brought downwards in an arc moving under the bars and up again to the surface of the water beyond the bars, followed by the trunk. The patient should then be in a supine position. The movement is then reversed bringing the legs and trunk back through the arc to the starting position. In this activity, resistance is given by the buoyancy of the water in the downward parts of the movements, and by increasing the speed of movement, resistance is also increased.

Exercises for Balance and Equilibrium Reactions

The Parkinson's disease patient will also benefit from exercises in water to improve the equilibrium reactions which are affected by this condition. The tilting reactions of the trunk and head are most commonly the responses which are affected first, and are generally more severely reduced than the other responses such as, propping reactions. Exercises which encourage these responses are described in the section of this chapter dealing with re-education of balance and equilibrium reactions (p. 79).

CONTRA-INDICATIONS TO HYDROTHERAPY

The following section lists possible contra-indications to hydrotherapy which pertain to the rehabilitation of neurological conditions. Where these conditions exist, hydrotherapy should not be included in the patient's programme.

● **Unstable blood pressure**

In the case of stroke patients with this problem or patients with conditions involving the autonomic control of blood pressure, the generalized heating of the body may cause a dramatic fall in blood pressure.

● **Cardiac conditions**

Many patients suffering from cerebrovascular disease may also have some cardio-vascular involvement, and the warmth of the pool water producing generalized heating of the body may place undue stress on the heart in order to maintain the blood pressure at normal levels.

● **Open wounds**

Patients with an open wound which is not small enough to be covered would be open to contracting infection from the pool; alternatively infection from a wound may be spread via the water to another patient.

● **Uncontrolled urinary incontinence**

This problem may be averted if the patient is involved in a bladder training programme, in which the bladder is regularly emptied by manual tapping and expressing or by intermittent catheterization. These procedures, performed immediately prior to the hydrotherapy session will allow many patients, otherwise ineligible for hydrotherapy, to participate in this therapy. For male patients, the problem can easily be solved by the use of urinary collection devices such as a urodome or catheter, which has been spigotted.

● **Bowel incontinence**

This is a problem to which no satisfactory remedy has been found.

● **Urinary and bowel tract infections**

The following conditions exclude the affected patients from the pool:

Methicillin resistant *Staphylococcus aureus*, diarrhoea or non diarrhoeal gastrointestinal infections, hepatitis A, non A non B hepatitis, vesicular skin conditions and patients with open or weeping lesions who are known or suspected to be carriers of blood borne diseases, e.g. hepatitis B or HIV.

There is no reason to exclude patients with urinary tract infections from the pool as most of these infections are caused by normal bowel organisms that do not pose any threat to other people.

- Severe loss of sensation

Patients whose condition results in severe loss of all sensory modalities, in particular that of proprioception, often suffer a disorientation effect in water, and also are unable to see where their limbs are under water.

- Multiple sclerosis

In many cases the hydrotherapy pool temperature is too high for these patients. Increase in body temperature causes a slowing of nerve conduction, and in multiple sclerosis patients in which conduction is already slowed due to demyelination, this has the effect of weakening muscles and causing an increase in tone, as well as severe fatigue in many patients. In the author's experience, a water temperature of around 32–33°C may be suitable for most of the patients with this condition, however, for some, it may still be too high.

ADVERSE REACTIONS

The physiotherapist should be aware of certain reactions which may occur during hydrotherapy treatment of some of the conditions mentioned earlier in this chapter. The signs which notify the physiotherapist that the medium is having an effect which is detrimental to the treatment aims or to the safety of the patient are listed below, and the physiotherapist must be alert to their appearance.

● **Increased tone**

This may be due to the patient's anxiety or fear of water, but teaching the skills necessary for mental adjustment and balance restoration may overcome fear (Reid Campion, 1985). It may also be due to a water temperature that is too high (Stockmeyer, 1967). In the author's experience excessive effort caused by too high a resistance may cause an increase in tone. Inappropriate handling may contribute to an increase of tone.

● **Nausea**

The water's action or turbulence may induce nausea due to vestibular stimulation in some patients with vestibular tract involvement (e.g. stroke and multiple sclerosis).

● **Cardio-vascular effects**

Signs of cardio-vascular distress can be evident by increased redness or pallor, excessive sweating and in increased respiratory rate. Patients having these symptoms should be quickly removed from the pool, and observations made of blood pressure and pulse rate, until these have normalized.

● **Breathing distress**

Breathing distress may occur in deeper water in those patients with very weak respiratory muscles. The water pressure can be strong enough in some cases to overcome the strength of these muscles and seriously inhibit thoracic expansion. In this event, the patient should be treated in shallow water, adopt the supine lying position with the chest clear of the water or in extreme cases removed from the pool.

● **Increased weakness**

The warmth of the water may, if too high in cases of multiple sclerosis or demyelinating diseases, cause slowing of nerve conduction velocity and increasing weakness of the patient's muscles.

● **Epilepsy**

Some stroke patients may be prone to fitting and the physiotherapist should be aware of this possibility.

● **Emergencies**

Physiotherapists and pool attendants must be fully conversant with resuscitation procedures for use in emergencies e.g. cardiac arrest, and be watchful for any indication of such an emergency occurring.

POINTS TO REMEMBER

To make a full and effective use of hydrotherapy in the total rehabilitation programme of neurological patients, there are certain principles which should be applied.

● The assessment of each patient on land should determine the need for treatment in the water, however, an assessment should also be made on the patient in water. This is because the ability of the patient will vary from that on land, and the aims and treatment will be varied accordingly.
● In the case of stroke patients, treatments generally should be on an individual basis, in order for the physiotherapist to be aware of any increase in tone or incorrect movement patterns, and to correct them immediately. The patient must not be allowed to practise movements which are incorrect as they can become habitual and very difficult to correct.
● Exercises in water are different from exercises on land due to the properties inherent in water, such as buoyancy and turbulence. Land-based exercises should not be used in water, as different conditions pertain, and the use of water's unique properties is important.
● Hydrotherapy should not be considered as a sole treatment in itself for the neurological patient, but part of a total rehabilitation programme. It should complement the other parts of a patient's programme, by working towards the goals which have been set, both by the patient, and by the rehabilitation team.

REFERENCES

Atkinson H.W. (1986). Aspects of neuro-anatomy and physiology. In *Cash's Textbook of Neurology for Physiotherapists* 4th edn. (Downie P.A. ed.) London: Faber & Faber.

Bobath B. (1978). *Adult Hemiplegia: Evaluation & Treatment* 2nd edn. Oxford: Heinemann Medical.

Brunnstrom S. (1970). *Movement Therapy in Hemiplegia: A Neurophysiological Approach*, New York: Harper and Row.

Caillet R. (1980). *The Shoulder in Hemiplegia*, Philadelphia: F.A. Davis Co.

Carr J., Shepherd R. (1982). *A Motor Learning Programme for Stroke*, Oxford: Heinemann Medical.

Franchimont P., Juchmers P., Lecomte J. (1983). Hydrotherapy—Mechanisms and Indications. *Pharmac. Therapy*, **20**.

Gossman M.R., Sahrmann S.A., Rose S.J. (1982). Review of Length Associated Changes in Muscle—Experimental Evidence and Clinical Implications. *Physical Therapy*, **62, 12**, 1799–1808.

Johnstone M. (1982). *The Stroke Patient—Principles of Rehabilitation*, Edinburgh: Churchill Livingstone.

Kaltenborn F.M. (1980). *Mobilization of the extremity joints: examination and basic treatment techniques.* 3rd edn. Oslo, Norway: Olaf Norlis Bokhandel.

Maitland G.D. (1977). *Peripheral Manipulation* 2nd edn. London: Butterworths.

Martin J. (1981). The Halliwick method, *Physiotherapy*, **67**.

Reid Campion M. (1985). *Hydrotherapy in Paediatrics*, Oxford; Heinemann Medical.

Skinner A.T., Thomson A.M. eds. (1983). *Duffield's Exercise in Water*, London: Ballière and Tindall.

Stockmeyer S. (1967). An Interpretation of the Approach of Rood to the Treatment of Neuromuscular Dysfunction, *American Journal of Physical Medicine*, **46**, 1.

5

Jane McGIBBON
Wendy ELFORD

Hydrotherapy in Spinal Cord Injuries

Hydrotherapy has proved to be an extremely useful modality in the rehabilitation of many neuromuscular conditions (Guttman, 1976) and spinal injuries are no exception.

Specific exercises and movement re-education form the basis of any rehabilitation programme. The physiotherapist can utilize the buoyancy and resistance provided by the water to attempt activities not possible on land. In addition, the swimming skills learned in hydrotherapy sessions will increase the patient's confidence and safety in water and enable participation in the many water sports now adapted for the disabled.

Hydrotherapy is therefore not only a useful addition to a formal rehabilitation programme but helps to provide a sound basis for future recreational skills.

In this chapter, two main treatment groups will be considered:

1. Spinal injuries with paralysis, either complete or incomplete.
2. Spinal injuries with no neurological deficit but with a significant vertebral fracture or fracture dislocation.

All patients with significant spinal fractures are treated by the spinal unit at the Royal Perth (Rehabilitation) Hospital where the authors have worked. Hence the inclusion here of patients without neurological deficit.

THE ADVANTAGES OF HYDROTHERAPY

Freedom of movement—the major advantage in treating spinal injured patients in the water is that they can have complete freedom of movement with total body support from very early in their rehabilitation programme. It is, however, advisable in the case of very unstable fractures to wait for six weeks or until some bony union is obvious before embarking on any hydrotherapy programme (Bedbrook and Donovan, 1982).

Elimination of gravity—the upright position is often unattainable in the early stages not only because of the paralysis, whether complete or incomplete, but because of non-union of the vertebral fracture. Patients immersed in water to the level of the neck have effectively only 8% of their body weight on their feet. This increases to approximately 50% at the level of the anterior superior iliac spine (ASIS) (Harrison and Bulstrode, 1987). This partial elimination of gravity in the upright position allows weight bearing through the legs from the very early stages of rehabilitation. Walking can also be commenced if there is sufficient innervation of trunk and low limb musculature.

Exercises many joints and muscles—exercise programmes using the water for assistance and resistance can be devised incorporating large numbers of joints and muscles.

Relief of pain—in some cases the warmth of the water will relieve pain and spasticity, leading to increased mobility, enjoyment and high morale.

Relief of pressure—pressure is relieved from bony prominences, for example the ischial tuberosities and malleoli (Turner, 1981).

There is a significant psychological benefit in being independent of a wheelchair and experiencing freedom of movement without the effects of gravity.

DISADVANTAGES AND PRECAUTIONS OF HYDROTHERAPY

Although the advantages far outweigh the disadvantages when exercising in water, there are a few disadvantages for which measures can be taken to minimize inconvenience and distress.

Respiratory distress—Complete tetraplegia results in the paralysis of the respiratory muscles of the thoracic cage. The diaphragm is also involved in lesions of C3–4. The pressure of water on the abdomen causes some resistance to breathing; this pressure can eventually be overcome and can be seen as a positive improvement in overall respiratory function.

Risks of water activity—any activity in water for both the able-bodied and disabled carries certain risks. The extreme risk is that of drowning, but for the disabled patient and especially the person suffering from a high spinal lesion, anxiety about this risk is paramount. For these people and for all disabled, constant supervision is essential, both from within the water and from the sides of the pool. For safety reasons all staff should be trained in resuscitation techniques. When a physiotherapist is conducting hydrotherapy programmes in the water it is vital that pool-side staff should consist of at least one nurse trained in resuscitation techniques and one nursing assistant similarly trained.

Incontinence—in the spinal cord injured patients, bladder and bowel function are frequently impaired. Bowel incontinence should not be tolerated in any hydrotherapy setting. Some urinary incontinence is acceptable in the non-infected patient (Pearman, 1987, personal communication), and those on strict fluid balance charts should wear a collection device (Riley, 1987, personal communication) (see also p. 66).

Temperature regulation—body temperature regulation of the patients should be watched carefully. All paraplegics above the level of T6 experience difficulties with temperature control (Guttman *et al.*, 1958; Guttman, 1970). This is evident in extremes of climate where tetraplegics manifest a body temperature close to the environmental reading over a long period. As vasomotor function adjusts, compensation occurs but never completely. Even after many years, patients may be extremely disturbed in extremes of temperature (Guttman *et al.*, 1958).

A water temperature of 32–34°C is desirable. Whilst overheating can occur in the water, sudden loss of body heat can also occur if the patient is left exposed for too long when out of the water. Ideally, patients should be removed quickly but safely from the water and immediately covered with towels or given a warm gown. They should then be dried and dressed before leaving the area.

The time spent on a swimming session varies with each patient's tolerance of the water temperature and the patient's general fitness. Patients at the Royal Perth (Rehabilitation) Hospital are advised to stay in the water for no longer than one hour, 30–45 min being the optimum time.

Ear problems and their management—during a hydrotherapy session, tetraplegics may spend a large amount of time floating on their backs with their ears under the water. A float around the neck, whilst lifting the head above the water level rarely prevents some water entering the ears. This combined with the relative immobility of tetraplegics when they are out of the water leads to an accumulation of water in the ear which can lead to inflammation. If water repellant drops or ear plugs are unsuccessful, routine drainage in the side lying position will decrease this risk.

THE AIMS OF TREATMENT FOR THE SPINAL INJURED PATIENT

The Neurologically Impaired Patient

The aims of treatment for the neurologically affected patient are not unlike those for other neurological conditions but there are some special considerations.

The isolation and strengthening of specific muscle groups

Any movement of a paraparetic limb whether performed voluntarily or not can provide the incentive needed to continue with an aggressive programme (Bromley, 1976). A muscle that may produce only a flicker of movement when out of the water can be positioned in the water so that, on contraction, it will give significant joint movement. This is advantageous to both the patient and physiotherapist as once there is movement a variety of exercise therapy techniques can then be employed.

Alleviation of spasticity

When treating a patient who shows excessive tone, it is important that this be inhibited as much as possible. The patient then has the sense of what is normal positioning and consequently can perform more normal movement patterns. Weak voluntary movement which is masked by spasticity can then be utilized.

It has been claimed that warm water decreases muscle tone in upper motor neuron lesions (Skinner and Thomson, 1983). This facilitates normal movement for the above reasons. In practice it is necessary to evaluate the effect of warm water on muscle tone in each individual patient where it is sufficiently increased to influence movement.

However, it is important to realize that overactivity can lead to fatigue in the muscles being exercised, the appearance of activity in other muscle groups via associated reactions and a movement of poorer quality.

To maintain or increase the range of movement of affected joints

Whenever possible, the physiotherapist must prevent a joint from stiffening and thereby saving the patient pain and the possibility of a permanent disability. Limitation of the range of movement impairs the function of a joint and the muscles that move it. Measures which increase the range of movement must therefore go hand in hand with those which build up sufficient muscle power to stabilize and control that movement.

Active exercise which leads to an increase in range, works the muscles and reminds the patient of the pattern of movement. It is the treatment of choice but in some cases passive and manipulative methods precede or assist its performance (Gardiner, 1971). These methods performed in the water are often diversional and of more interest to the patient which makes it a valuable adjunct to more localized treatments.

To offer overall mobility

A spinal injured person can usually only utilize two positions in order to be safe from falling and injuring himself. These are lying and sitting.

The support offered by water to all movements will lead to a freedom of movement not possible on land. Whether this freedom of movement is utilized to its full extent depends largely on the trust a patient develops with the physiotherapist and consequently his confidence in the water. Once this has been achieved, the freedom of movement gained will lead to an independence not possible on land.

To safely attain the upright position

The majority of spinally injured patients are routinely stood in the water. Most will report a feeling of well-being while in this position. This feeling of well-being particularly in the upper motor neuron lesions could be attributed to a general decrease in the muscle tone over the whole body. The achilles tendon has long been noted as a 'trigger point' in relation to spasticity. That is, it can be responsible for either increasing or decreasing spasticity depending on its position, the length of the tendon and how much weight is being transferred through it. The upright position gives both stretch and weight bearing to this tendon.

Standing also has the advantages of stretching the hip flexor and abdominal muscles that have been shortened through wheelchair sitting, aids in the control of postural hypotension and gives a start to ambulation (Michaelis, 1976) (Fig. 5.1).

To increase general fitness

As skills develop and a form of swimming is taught, cardio-vascular fitness and the endurance of innervated muscles will improve.

To promote socialization

Whether the pool sessions are used for specific exercises, competition or water games, socialization and interaction with both disabled and able-bodied people is consequential.

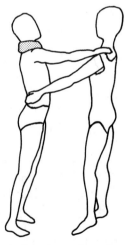

Fig. 5.1 Standing the spinal patient where knee stabilization is not required

Neurologically Intact Patient

The patient with a significant spinal fracture or fracture dislocation without neurological impairment can be exercised effectively in the water. Aims of treatment include the following:

Strengthening of spinal musculature

Whether there has been any surgical intervention of the neurologically intact patient or not, the erector spinae muscles always become weaker following a vertebral fracture (Kakulas, 1981). This weakness is exacerbated by the prolonged bedrest required to achieve postural reduction and healing of the fracture not suited to internal fixation.

Strengthening of the erector spinae muscles can be achieved easily in the comfort of warm water without placing undue strain on the vertebral column.

This form of exercise can continue unsupervised outside the rehabilitation centre. As these patients are often discharged early after mobilization, this has obvious advantages.

Reduction of muscle spasm, pain and stiffness

The protective muscle spasm contributing to pain and stiffness will also relax (Toth, 1983) and as strength and mobility increase, so will cardio-vascular fitness.

HYDROTHERAPY TECHNIQUES

Neurologically Impaired Spinal Patient

Hydrotherapy techniques suitable for a particular patient will depend on the level and completeness of the spinal cord injury. Complicating factors such as other injuries, limited joint range and the presence of spasticity must also be considered.

Before commencing hydrotherapy, it is advisable to confirm with medical staff which type of bracing is required or alternatively which spinal movements are to be avoided. Nursing staff will provide up-to-date information on the skin condition, and bowel control and the presence of any bladder infection which may prevent the patient attending the pool.

Table 5.1 Levels of innervation in tetraplegia. Formulated by W. Elford from a compilation by Kendall and McCreary (1983) with reference to Warwick and Williams (1973). Note: '?' denotes possible innervation at this level.

Last intact spinal level	Muscles innervated	Function
C4	Diaphragm	Respiration
	Sternocleidomastoid	Neck rotation, side flexion
	Rhomboids	Scapular retraction, elevation
C5	Deltoid	Shoulder abduction, horizontal flexion & extension
	Supraspinatus	Shoulder abduction
	Infraspinatus, Teres Minor	Shoulder external rotation
	Subscapularis	Shoulder internal rotation (weak)
	Pec. Major (clav. head)	Shoulder horizontal flexion (weak)
	Biceps, Brachialis, Brachioradialis	Elbow flexion
	? Supinator, ECRL, ECRB	See C6
C6	Pectoralis Major	Shoulder adduction, internal rotation
	Coracobrachialis	Shoulder flexion, adduction
	Teres Major	Shoulder internal rotation, extension, adduction
	Latissimus Dorsi	Scapular depression (weak), shoulder extension, internal rotation, adduction
	ECRL, ECRB	Radial wrist extension
	Supinator	Supination
	Pronator Teres	Pronation
	?Triceps, FCR	See C7
C7	Triceps	Elbow extension
	Flexor Carpi Radialis	Wrist flexion
	Extensor Digitorum	Finger extension (weak)
	Flexor Digitorum Superficialis	Finger MCP flexion (weak)
C8, T1	Flexor Digitorum Profundus	Finger IPJ flexion
	Intrinsics	Fine hand movements

High cervical lesions

It can be seen that patients with lesions above C6 have an imbalance between abduction and adduction and also external and internal rotation of the shoulder. Due to the absence of triceps, the arm can only be used as a short lever during swimming and exercise unless the elbow is locked passively. Out of the water, gravity will aid elbow extension if the shoulder is externally rotated and biceps inhibited. The resistance provided by the water will also passively extend the elbow during internal rotation and adduction or external rotation and abduction. Elbow flexion must, however be less than ninety degrees.

The patient with a C5 lesion will find it difficult to roll from prone to supine. Independent swimming may only be practical in supine, the prone position being used with direct supervision and assistance if the patient is unable to roll.

Low cervical lesions

Lesions of C7 or below leave sufficient innervation of shoulder musculature and triceps to allow a greater range of exercise and swimming options. The patient should be able to roll from prone to supine, making freestyle and breast stroke possible.

Wrist flexion, functional thumb and finger flexion and extension and intrinsics, if present, allow more effective use of the hand to push against the water. This improves propulsion. Webbed gloves may be of some assistance.

Mid cervical lesions

The patient with some innervation of C6 will fall somewhere between the two above groups in his abilities in the water. Here the patient's pre-injury waterskills and confidence, his determination and the quality and frequency of his instruction are of major importance in the achievement of maximum independence in the water.

Buoyancy and flotation for the tetraplegic

Buoyancy varies between individuals in the normal population. There are also differences in the buoyancy of individual segments of the body. If the specific gravity of the body or part of it is less than

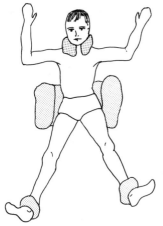

Fig. 5.2 An example of flotation for the spinal injured patient

one, it will float, if greater than one it will sink (Davis and Harrison, 1988). A low buoyancy will increase the need for flotation devices for safety. The normal individual uses upper and lower limb strength to push the head to the surface during swimming—the tetraplegic patient cannot always achieve this. Maximum flotation is advisable initially and also when the patient, especially those with low buoyancy, is not under close supervision. A neck collar, a firmly fitting pelvic float and an ankle float can be used (Fig 5.2).

Once the patient's buoyancy needs, confidence and safety have been evaluated, the foot and pelvic floats can be removed. It is important to note that feet dragging along the bottom of the pool may cause skin damage, in which case the ankle float should be replaced or socks worn for protection. Even competent disabled swimmers may choose to use an ankle float routinely.

Early water activity

Before commencing a more formal hydrotherapy programme, the tetraplegic patient must learn to maintain a safe, stable floating position in supine. Two key factors influence this. The amount of neck flexion or extension in relation to the trunk controls vertical rotation. Any asymmetry between the right and left sides of the body in shape and density will cause lateral rotation.

The patient must be able to control rotation in these two directions to be considered safe in the water with or without flotation during exercise and swimming activities. Maximum neck extension is essential to maintain a stable floating position in supine and is emphasized from the beginning. The patient must experience the consequences of failure to do this with minimal flotation early in his treatment. The patient in a cervical brace will have a static neck position and will require at least neck and pelvic floats. Control of lateral rotation can be taught by asking the patient to lift one arm slightly out of the water. Turning the head to the opposite side and sculling with the free arm will help to correct the rotation towards the lifted arm. Shoulder girdle retraction and shoulder extension on the opposite side also correct lateral rotation.

The more able patient with sufficient confidence could progress to rotation through 180° and 360°. From prone, rotation of the neck to one side with full retraction and extension of that shoulder and sculling movements of either or both arms will facilitate rolling. Alternatively the patient can be taught to use the gutter or bar at the side of the pool to right himself.

Before attempting rolling, some patients will require time in a supported sitting position getting accustomed to immersion of the face in a position they can control.

Exercise

At this stage, specific upper limb exercises can be introduced. The Bad Ragaz Ring Method (Skinner and Thomson, 1983; Davis and Harrison, 1988) can be used effectively to exercise the large muscle groups of the shoulder and elbow. Suitable patterns include isotonic single arm abduction, bilateral arm external rotation and finally, bilateral adduction and internal rotation.

Weak shoulder abductors and adductors can be strengthened isometrically by asking the patient to maintain a static position of the shoulder while being pushed and pulled through the water in supine. Patients with good wrist control and some hand function can use hand-held bats (possibly with straps) or floats for resisted upper limb exercise in the supine or sitting positions. The patient can be placed in an unsupported sitting position at or below shoulder depth to work on sitting balance. Standing at the edge of the pool or in open water with the support of the physiotherapist is also beneficial. Passive movements and muscle stretches for the limbs and trunk can also be performed in a supported position e.g. on a plinth.

Swimming

The simplest swimming activity is a modified backstroke. Both arms are abducted together, moving through or slightly lifted from the water, and then pulled to the side. If there is an imbalance between the strength of the abductors and the adductors, there will be a tendency to use mid-range only, because the weaker adductors are disadvantaged by working in the outer range.

Some adduction of the shoulder is necessary to achieve a functional stroke. Following the stroke through underneath the pelvis will help to compensate for low buoyancy. Some patients may have difficulty maintaining passive elbow extension without triceps, particularly if biceps are overactive. Patients with asymmetrical lesions will experience difficulty in maintaining a straight course. This can be overcome with practice by reducing the power of the stroke on the stronger side or by using the head as a rudder, side flexing it towards the strong side.

The patient with low buoyancy and those who use vigorous strokes will tend to become submerged even when full neck extension is maintained. This will also happen if both arms are lifted right out of the water due to the effect of the metacentric principle.

Maintaining full inflation of the lungs for the greatest part of each stroke is vital. Rapid inspiration and expiration should occur at the end of one stroke before commencing the next to maintain optimum buoyancy. The more active patient may become totally submerged temporarily but will return to the surface—accurate timing of breathing is essential. A diving mask is useful at this stage to protect the patient's eyes and nose allowing concentration on neck extension and breathing.

Swimming activities in prone are only advisable in the patient who is confident and can roll from prone to a safe position in supine unaided. Direct supervision with assistance for rolling using a pre-arranged signal can be used. It is possible to introduce snorkelling in less able patients with maximum supervision and assistance. Scuba equipment is even used in some rehabilitation centres (U. Stahli, 1988; personal communication). More buoyant patients will find that flotation of the pelvis and legs in prone will actually make it more difficult to get the head sufficiently clear of the water to take a breath. However, some more able swimmers choose to use an ankle float when training. The mid to low level tetraplegic patient can achieve freestyle, breaststroke and butterfly

(Carlson, 1982). There may be difficulty attaining enough extension, external rotation and abduction to get arm recovery in freestyle. Poor neck and upper body rotation may cause problems in incorporating lateral breathing. Some patients almost roll to supine to take a breath. In breaststroke, propulsion is achieved by strong internal rotation and depression. External rotation and flexion of the shoulder during the recovery stroke will also produce passive elbow extension. Strong shoulder depressors and directing the stroke underneath the body will help to push the head to the surface for a breath.

Incomplete tetraplegia

Patients with incomplete lesions, especially those with some sparing of lower limb and trunk musculature will also require a specific programme for these muscles. Early gait re-education if possible can be achieved in the water and activities in standing work towards this. Stabilizing the patient on a submerged plinth or weighted chair can provide the opportunity for vigorous exercise under less supervision.

The body asymmetry resulting from the incomplete lesion will provide difficulties in maintaining lateral rotation stability and a straight course in supine or prone swimming. This is offset by the advantage of a greater number of innervated muscles and can be overcome with training.

Paraplegia

Upper limb strengthening, trunk strengthening where possible and swimming activities form the basic treatment of the paraplegic patient. If spinal bracing is required in the pool initially, strengthening of the trunk will be limited to isometric exercise. This can be achieved with strongly resisted upper limb exercises using hand-held bats or floats. Alternatively, exercises where the trunk is moved through the water with the arms providing anchorage on the side of the pool or plinth are effective.

Once the brace is removed, the range of static and dynamic exercises can be increased. Bad Ragaz techniques including trunk stabilization in float support supine lying can be used to strengthen the trunk muscles. The physiotherapist stands between the patient's legs stabilizing the pelvis and moves the patient in an arc through the water. The patient must maintain a static position of the trunk against the resistance of the water. As a progression, the patient side-flexes in the direction of movement.

Balance and strength of spinal musculature can be improved by exercise in a sitting position. Initially, the patient may sit on the physiotherapist's knee or on a weighted chair or step. The arms should be forwards to maintain balance, and the hips, knees and ankles as near a right angle as can be achieved. Turbulence is used to stress the patient's balance in these positions. More capable patients can 'sit' without a chair (see page 52). This demands considerable balance control and muscle work. With the physiotherapist providing pelvic fixation, the patient can perform trunk flexion and combined flexion/rotation or simply try to maintain an erect posture while the physiotherapist moves the patient in all directions through the water or creates turbulence around the body. Isotonic and isometric trunk flexion and extension can also be done in side lying using the same basic technique. If the patient was formerly a strong swimmer, little instruction should be needed. Buoyancy and the patient's ability to recover from prone should be examined initially and pelvic or foot floats provided if necessary. The patient should swim only with supervision at first.

Incomplete paraplegia and cauda equina lesions

In patients with incomplete or low level paraplegia, a specific strengthening programme for innervated muscles will be required (see Table 5.2 for levels of innervation). There are numerous exercises described in the chapter on orthopaedic injuries suitable for strengthening lower limb musculature. These will therefore, not be listed here (see Chapter 00). Davis and Harrison (1988) also describe the Bad Ragaz patterns for the lower limb in detail. Patterns are selected according to the level of innervation as there will be imbalances between muscle groups e.g. abductors and adductors.

Early gait retraining may be possible even with minimal muscle strength. The depth of water in which this is attempted is critical as joint control is impaired where muscles are weak and sensation poor in a buoyancy dominated situation. However, in shallower water, the innervated muscles may be too weak to support the body's weight. Commencing gait training with the patient immersed to just below the axilla is suggested.

Any orthosis required for ambulation, for example an ankle foot orthosis, can be adapted for use in the pool.

Table 5.2   Levels of innervation in paraplegia. Formulated by W. Elford from a compilation by Kendall and McCreary (1983) with reference to Warwick and Williams (1973).

Last spinal level intact	Muscles innervated	Function
T1 & below	Erector Spinae	Spinal extension
T(7),8 & below	Abdominals	Spinal flexion
T12	Quadratus Lumborum	Pelvic elevation
L2	Psoas Major	Hip flexion
	Sartorius	Hip flexion, external rotation, Knee flexion
	Quadriceps	Knee extension
	Adductor group	Hip adduction
L3	Obturator Externus	Hip external rotation, adduction
L4–5	Gluteus Minimus, Tensor Fasciae Latae	Hip internal, abduction
	Gluteus Medius	Hip abduction
	Gemelli, Obturator Internus	Hip external rotation, abduction
	Quadratus Femoris	Hip external rotation
	Anterior Tibial Group	Ankle dorsiflexion, inversion
L5	Hamstrings	Knee flexion, Hip extension
	Gluteus Maximus	Hip extension
	Peronei	Ankle eversion
S1	Posterior Tibial Group	Ankle plantarflexion

Recreation

In addition to a more formal exercise programme in the hydrotherapy pool, games and watersports tailored to the abilities of the individual or group can be a great success.

Snorkelling with the supervision of the physiotherapist is a possibility for the less able tetraplegics who are unable to roll independently. Scuba equipment is even used in some rehabilitation centres where the staff have the skills and adapted equipment available (Stahli, 1988; personal communication). Specialized flotation equipment can be used to support the paralysed patient in a vertical position so that he can participate in ball games such as water polo. One example of these—'Wetvests'—are made of

Neoprene rubber with extra flotation added (J. Thompson, 1989; personal communication).

If poolside and therapy staff are vigilant, such equipment increases the safety and confidence of patients, making group games more practical and enjoyable. There are many water sports adapted for the disabled such as rowing, sailing surfcatting and waterskiing. All of these require the disabled person to have a minimum level of water skills. Early exposure to these sports as a spectator and encouragement with swimming skills will help to broaden recreation opportunities for these people in the community.

The Neurologically Intact Patient

Trunk strengthening exercises, particularly those emphasizing extension are an important part of the hydrotherapy programme for the neurologically intact patient. Hyperflexion is a common mechanism of injury and strong back extensors will help to protect the spine from deformity once bracing is removed.

Exercises requiring static trunk work are commenced early while the patient still requires bracing. This can be achieved with a combination of formal exercises and swimming.

Early exercises

- float resisted hip extension, supine lying on the plinth
- alternate straight leg kicking, supine lying
- static trunk strengthening in float support supine lying (see p. 116)
- standing—small range, hip flexion/extension and abduction adduction
- standing—bilateral shoulder flexion/extension and abduction adduction resisted by hand-held bats
- backwards walking
- sideways walking
- backstroke

Progression of exercises

Once bracing is no longer required and the patient is allowed to commence gentle active mobilization the following exercises may be gradually added.

- bilateral leg movements side to side in supine lying on the plinth
- bilateral buoyancy resisted hip and trunk flexion and assisted extension prone lying on the plinth
- trunk side flexion and rotation (reversed origin) in a vertical elbow support position at the end of the plinth. Knees and hips are flexed; the pelvis is tilted laterally or rotated.
- float resisted hip and back extension in supine lying
- bilateral float or physiotherapist resisted trunk extension and rotation in float support supine lying
- isotonic trunk side flexion in float support supine lying
- freestyle and breaststroke may be added when back extension is sufficient.

The patient will be able to continue many of these exercises at his local pool after discharge.

Methods of Entering and Leaving the Pool

Ideally all pools in rehabilitation centres should have a hoist incorporating a plinth or chair carrying system. The plinth should have an adjustable section to cater for the supine or semi-reclined patient. Some spinal injured patients, particularly the lower level paraplegics can be taught to enter and leave the pool independently transferring to and from their wheelchairs, but age, the level of the lesion and their general fitness together with the structure of the surrounding walls of the pool are some of the limiting factors.

The usual method is to transfer from the wheelchair to the ground allowing the buttocks to slip forward over the edge of the chair, and then carefully to the side of the pool provided this is level with the floor. Once at the edge the patient can fall forwards or sideways into the water or lower gently into the water legs first using the same method as for leaving the wheelchair. Some pools have a small wall incorporated into the surrounds which if at wheelchair height, eliminates the need to transfer down to the ground.

Leaving the pool independently requires a lot of strength but is achieved by facing the side of the pool, placing both hands palms down on the edge and lifting the body up to the height whereby the buttocks can be turned and placed on the edge. The legs can then be lifted out and the patient can move to his chair and transfer into it using his preferred method.

Patients who are unable to lift themselves directly out of the pool using the above method may be able to use the step ladder at one end of the pool. A towel over the pool edge is necessary to protect the skin. The patient then carefully pulls himself over the edge of the pool using the rails. Should no hoist be available or the patient is unable to transfer independently, hydrotherapy is still possible if help is available to lift the patient to the side, and in and out of the water. This is strenuous work and a drain on man-power when in a hospital setting, but after discharge, family members and friends may make a swimming session possible. If a patient needs to be removed quickly from the water for reasons such as acute chest pain, anxiety or an impending bowel action, he should be floated to the side and lifted out using the nursing staff and pool attendants.

REFERENCES

Bedbrook G. M., Donovan W. W. (1982). Spinal Cord Injury. *Clinical Symposia* **34**(2), 2–36.

Bromley (1976). *Tetraplegia and Paraplegia. A guide for Physiotherapists.* London: Churchill Livingstone.

Carlson P. (1982). *Adaptive Techniques for Therapeutic Swimming,* (United States); Marianjoy Rehabilitation Hospital (Video cassette).

Davis B., Harrison R. (1988). *Hydrotherapy in Practice,* Edinburgh: Churchill Livingstone.

Gardiner M. D. (1971). *The Principles of Exercise Therapy* 3rd edn. London: G. Bell & Son.

Guttman L. (1970). Spinal Shock and Reflex Behaviour in Man. *Paraplegia* **8**, p. 100–116.

Guttman L. (1976). *Textbook of Sports for the Disabled.* Aylesbury: H.M. & M. Publisers.

Guttman L., Silver J., Wyndham C. H. (1958). Thermoregulation in spinal man. *Journal of Physiology* **142**, 406–419.

Harrison R., Bulstrode S. (1987). Percentage Weight Bearing During Partial Immersion in the Hydrotherapy Pool. *Physiotherapy Practice*, **3**, 60–63.

Kakulas B. S. (1981). Pathologic considerations of spinal paralysis. In (Bedrook G. M. ed.) *The Care and Management of Spinal Cord Injuries.* New York: Springer Verlag.

Kendall H. O., Kendall F. P., McCreary E. K. (1983) *Muscles: Testing and Function.* Baltimore: Williams and Wilkins.

Michaelis, L. S. (1976). Spasticity in spinal cord injuries. In *Handbook of*

Clinical Neurology, (Vinken P. J., Bruyn, G. W. eds.) **26**, p. 447–487, Amsterdam: North Holland.

Skinner A. T., Thomson A. M. (1983). *Duffield's Exercise in Water* (3rd edn.) London: Baillière Tindall.

Toth L. L. (1983). Spasticity management in spinal cord injury. *Rehabilitation Nursing* **8(1)**, 14–17.

Turner A. (1981). Decubiti, In *Lifetime Care of the Paraplegic Patient.* (Bedbrook G.M. ed.) pp 54–66, London: Churchill Livingstone.

Williams P. L., Warwick R. (1980). *Gray's Anatomy* (36th edn.). London: Churchill Livingstone.

FURTHER READING

Farrell F.T. (1976). A hydrotherapy programme for high cervical cord lesions. *Physiotherapy Canada*, **28(1)**, 9–12.

6

LYNETTE M. TINSLEY
BEVERLEY LAING

Hydrotherapy in Rheumatic Disease and Fibrositis

INTRODUCTION

In this chapter, consideration will be given to a variety of rheumatic conditions under the following headings:

Inflammatory arthritis ⎫
Degenerative arthritis ⎬ (Lynette M. Tinsley)
Spondyloarthropathies ⎭
Fibrositis (Beverley Laing)

ADVANTAGES OF HYDROTHERAPY

The advantages of hydrotherapy for rheumatic conditions are similar to those for all conditions. Of particular value are the warmth of the water which decreases pain and muscle spasm, while buoyancy relieves the stresses on joints especially those involved in weight bearing.

Assessment and Planning of Treatment

For each of the categories given above, the person should be individually assessed both subjectively and objectively (see p. 13). The assessment will help to establish the patient's needs, aims of treatment, realistic goals of treatment and treatment priorities (Harrison, 1980). In rheumatic diseases alterations in shape and density are as relevant to a water activity programme as in any other condition (Chapter 1).

Clinical signs and symptoms in rheumatic disorders

Common clinical signs and symptoms in the rheumatic disorders are pain occurring in and around affected joints, creating tension and muscle spasm; decreased range of motion and increased stiffness of joints; muscle weakness; deformities in some conditions and diminished functional ability.

Contra-indications

The contra-indications of hydrotherapy for the rheumatic disorders are common to all pool users: cardiac or respiratory failure, infective skin conditions including tinea pedis, excessively low, high or uncontrolled blood pressure, active TB, urinary infections, urinary or faecal incontinence and morbid hydrophobia (Atkinson and Harrison, 1981; Golland, 1981) (see also pp 66 and 99).

There are no contra-indications peculiar to the rheumatic diseases patient, except for those people in the early stages of recovery from a generalized flare of rheumatoid arthritis, when over activity or exertion could cause a recurrence of the symptoms of pain and swelling. Abnormal physiological measurements, for example, altered blood pressure or diminished vital capacity, should form no barrier to the person participating in hydrotherapy, providing the condition is recognized and monitored (Harrison, 1980; Harrison, 1981). Occasionally, a patient will complain of hypersensitive skin reacting to the chlorine. This may be a drug-induced reaction. A person with a single inflamed joint need not be excluded from the pool provided the affected joint is adequately restrained by a splint. Plastazote thermoplastic splinting material can be used but for the very frail, an alternative material or weighting of the splint may be necessary due to the increased buoyancy created by the splint. Similarly, a cervical collar of moulded Plastazote can be used for those people with cervical spine involvement, this can be individually moulded or commercially manufactured.

Whilst not being a contra-indication to hydrotherapy, a person with *osteoporosis* should be treated with caution, bearing in mind that even a slight degree of over exertion or sudden movement can lead to fractures.

As well as hydrotherapy, the patient should be encouraged to participate in weight bearing exercises to stimulate the bone, as there seems to be little evidence from scientific studies on the effect of exercising in water and the effect of other non-weight bearing exercises on bone density. Recent research indicates that bone density is increased by swimming (Orwoll *et al.*, 1987).

Exercise in water provides a safe environment for exercising and for the severe osteoporotic, may be the only safe exercise medium.

Primary aims of treatment

The primary aims of treatment for most rheumatic conditions are:

- relief of pain, swelling and stiffness
- promotion of relaxation
- joint mobilization
- muscle strengthening
- correction/prevention of contractures
- improvement of coordination and functional ability
- improvement of morale

INFLAMMATORY ARTHRITIS

Rheumatoid arthritis is a systemic, inflammatory disorder characteristically involving peripheral joints, often symmetrically. It can also manifest itself in other tissues and organs for example, the heart, lungs, eyes or nervous system. Weight loss, fever, depression, altered functional abilities and body shape and frequently, poor self esteem are common features.

Aims of Treatment

The aims of treatment for inflammatory disorders are:

- relief of pain and muscle spasm
- maintenance or restoration of muscle strength
- reduction of deformities and increased range of motion of all affected joints; the stretching of contractures, maintenance of range of motion and muscle power around unaffected joints
- promotion of relaxation
- re-education of correct walking patterns
- improvement of functional abilities and morale (Golland, 1981; Reid Campion, 1985).

Water temperature

In the author's experience, a water temperature of 35°C is that of choice (see also p. 9). Patients immersed in warm water should be carefully observed for adverse reactions and where these occur appropriate action should be taken.

Procedure Prior to an Exercise Programme

Following the initial assessment on land, and the decision to provide a water activity programme, the patient should be prepared for the procedure. The physiotherapist should describe the pool, the mode of transport from the ward to the pool, the method of entry into the water, an outline of what is expected of the patient and the type of activity to be carried out. If the analysis of the patient's shape and/or density has shown alteration which may produce rotational effects of the body when in the water these can also be explained to the patient who can be given instructions as to how to control these patterns when they occur. Thus the person is prepared for hydrotherapy and any apprehension diminished.

Safety

Safety procedures are not different for the rheumatic disease patient. The same principles apply as for all patients undertaking hydrotherapy treatment (Martin, 1981; Campion 1983; Reid Campion, 1985). The initial assessment will determine the person's capabilities and suitability for either individual or group treatment.

Individual programme

It is advisable, whenever possible, to conduct the earliest treatments on an individual basis for a short duration of time. Five to ten minutes to begin with gradually increasing the length of time. The emphasis of the treatment should be on relaxation, gentle movements and controlled stretching.

Technique

Method of entry and introduction to water

The technique of entry into the pool at this early stage is in most cases by mechanical hoist to diminish activity and stress on affected joints if recovering from a recent flare (see p. 124). Once in the water, the person is either positioned on a plinth in support lying, held in head support lying by the physiotherapist or in float support lying for the exercises. An apprehensive person may well be less concerned if allowed to stand in the deeper water holding onto the grab rail, with the physiotherapist nearby, for a period of time, until they are confident in water; or they may sit on a weighted chair, strapped in and instructed to keep the head forward to maintain the upright sitting position. Mentally adjusting the patient to the element of water and teaching balance restoration will help to overcome any problems of apprehension—see p. 17. Early exercise can begin with relaxation using gentle active, sweeping movements within a pain-free range the patient limiting the movement and breathing exercises, until the person feels relaxed and confident in the water. Once confidence is gained, more formalized exercises can be introduced for mobilizing and strengthening. Again, the Halliwick means of blowing to keep the nose and mouth clear of water should be taught.

Mobilization

The movement of acute or very painful joints should be avoided and care should be taken not to over-stretch peri-articular structures during joint mobilization. This can easily occur in a pool due to the difficulty with fixation and isolation of movement of a specific joint. The physiotherapist must therefore, control the amount of activity during the exercise, or ensure isolation of movement by the use of appropriate floats. Techniques which can be employed for joint mobilization are: *Bad Ragaz patterns* which use mass movement of the limbs and the trunk, isotonically, or isometrically, (Davis, 1967; Davis, 1971; Skinner and Thomson, 1983). Uncontrolled stretchings should be avoided to prevent damage to peri-articular structures and an increase of the inflammatory process, therefore, modification of the techniques, either by alteration of grip or limitation of range of motion, may be necessary (Harrison, 1980).

Hold–relax techniques—in some instances hold–relax techniques can be used to improve range of motion of a joint where muscle spasm is the limiting factor. In water the position of the patient is important so that buoyancy assists movement in the required direction. They are valuable techniques useful in the treatment of ankylosing spondylitis (Barefoot—Lecture notes, 1988).

Strengthening

Muscle strengthening around a painful joint

Muscle strengthening requires care. A method of achieving this is by the use of stabilizations or isometric contractions, whereby the physiotherapist puts the joint into a pain-free position and holds distally to the joint. The patient 'holds' the position whilst the physiotherapist moves the patient in different directions, causing different muscle groups to contract. Range of movement is gradually reduced and the direction of movement changed more quickly, giving rise to co-contraction of muscles around the joint. This method prevents stress on the joint, but allows for an increase of resistance.

Muscle strengthening can be achieved by the use of finely graded exercises using buoyancy as assistance, support or resistance; turbulence whereby resistance can be given either by increasing the speed of movement, altering the length of the lever arm or by using equipment such as floats or bats, which can be used to streamline or unstreamline and thus alter the resistance to movement. A narrow surface offers little resistance, a flat surface increases the resistance. Bad Ragaz techniques of mass patterns of movement using those patterns which counteract deformity and move pain-free joints can also be used for muscle strengthening.

When using floats as a resistance to a movement, the amount of resistance represented should be known. To prevent further damage to a joint, the person should have sufficient control over the active elements of the exercises (buoyancy resistance and assistance) and the return to the starting positions.

As a guideline to the amount of resistance provided by a float, a 3 in cube of polystyrene requires 1 lb of pressure to submerge it (Harrison, 1980). At all times, care must be taken to prevent stress on an already compromised joint, for example, the lever arm may need to be shortened in the exercise abduction of the hip and the resistance may need to be given over the knee joint rather than at the ankle (Skinner and Thomson, 1983).

Group Treatments

It may be necessary, due to large patient numbers and restricted staff levels in many departments and hospitals, to conduct treatments as a group rather than individually. As soon as practical after the initial introductory treatment, the patient should be included into a group activity. A general programme of exercises is given as a toning workout incorporating warm-up, mobility, strengthening exercises, breathing exercises, posture awareness and patient education. Time is allowed at the end of the session for attention to the specific needs of the individual. To participate in a group activity, patients should be confident in the water and at least semi-independent. Ideally, the group should be made up of those with similar disabilities, but as this is rarely the case, the physiotherapist must be prepared to conduct a session in which participants may be in the starting positions of lying, sitting or standing, so the exercises will need to be modified according to the restrictions placed on the individual by the apparatus.

Advantages

The advantages of group activity are encouragement, stimulation, motivation and social interaction, which occur whilst working with people with similar disabilities.

Disadvantages

Certain disadvantages can be experienced when working in groups. These are related to the size of the group, the positioning of group members and the physiotherapist, the size, shape and depth of the pool and the ability of the physiotherapist to safely provide adequate control and supervision of the exercises. Too large a group may make positioning the group members in the appropriate depths difficult, in that the group may become too widely spread for adequate control of safety and accurate supervision of exercise performance. This is particularly so where the pool is larger. However, a smaller pool, especially one where the depth is the same, poses the problem of positioning group members in appropriate depths.

Further difficulties arise within a group situation where visual and auditory problems exist amongst the participants. Distractions within the group itself and movements around the pool area can add to difficulty of the physiotherapist's task. The number of participants should be limited, preferably to 8–10, provided most people are able to maintain their balance and feel reasonably confident in water. Positioning within the pool should enable the physiotherapist to be within easy reach of each person for correction of the exercises or in the event of patients experiencing difficulties.

The Role of Education

The treatment time spent in the pool can be utilized as an important education period, creating body awareness and promoting the principles of joint preservation and work simplification. For example, during exercises for the hands, the physiotherapist can emphasize the stresses placed on wrist and meta-carpophalangeal joints during activities of daily living, such as dusting, turning taps and opening of jars. Alternative ways to perform these tasks can be suggested to prevent ulnar drift and strain on the joint. Whilst performing an exercise, explanation of the specific joint movement involved can highlight the importance of the activity, for example, internal rotation and adduction of the shoulder, to put the hands behind the back is an important movement required for toileting. A further example is the importance of strong quadriceps muscles to maintain stability of the knee and to facilitate walking, getting in and out of chairs, or walking up and down stairs. The importance of correct postural habits can be related to their effect on body mechanics. Explaining simply the functional activity of an exercise and the muscles involved in the performance of the action can give a greater understanding of the importance of the exercises.

As part of the education process it is useful to ask the patient to select an exercise and for them to explain the reason for the exercise, which muscles are working and thus the functional activity of the movement involved in, for example opening doors, hanging up clothes and walking. Performance of the exercises should be slow, gentle and non stressful. Gentle exercise is emphasized as opposed to vigorous. Many people tend to believe that the harder they work the more beneficial it is, whereas if practised, there is a greater likelihood of further damage.

Exercise Programmes for Patients with Inflammatory Arthritis

In the case of the person with inflammatory arthritis, the exercises will be modified according to the individual's abilities and disabilities. There will also be variation between the programmes selected for individual treatments and group treatments.

Individual treatments

Individual treatments are usually given for the sub-acute and immediate post-acute phases. The initial sessions can be from 5–

10 min, gradually progressing in time according to the patient's tolerance. Exercises are commenced as non-weight bearing exercises, concentrating on relaxation techniques and large functional movements.

Relaxation

Relaxation can be practised with the person floating, using the effect of buoyancy. Support can be given by the use of floats around the neck and hips and possibly the ankles. In the supine floating position, the person can be encouraged to breathe deeply, to tense muscles and relax them and to consciously allow the body to be supported by the buoyancy of the water. Imagery, such as imagining oneself floating in a peaceful environment, may be used. To promote relaxation, the physiotherapist can sweep the lower limbs and trunk from side to side slowly and rhythmically through the water. The hold should be at the centre of balance of the body, approximately waist level, thus giving the physiotherapist maximum control and the person a feeling of security.

Modification of this hold may be necessary where a large or tall person presents a problem. The physiotherapist will need to take the hands nearer the hips to achieve the swinging movement easily. To achieve this hold the person's neck should rest on one of the physiotherapist's shoulders which has been lowered slightly to allow the head to pass over the shoulder.

Mobilizing and Strengthening Exercises

Mobilizing and strengthening exercises can be carried out in flotation on a one-to-one basis but care must be taken to prevent over stretching of peri-articular structures (see p. 127). The physiotherapist must be able to control the amount of activity, to isolate the movements with adequate fixation and to be aware of the amount of resistance by the floats when used. The patient should be able to control the active element of the exercise and the return to the starting position (Harrison, 1980).

Mobilizing exercises—can be active assisted movements, hold–relax techniques, active sweeping movements or pattern movements e.g. for the shoulder joint the flexion-abduction lateral rotation pattern; for the knee single or double knee flexions patterns.

Strengthening exercises—around a painful joint can be achieved by isometric contractions or stabilizations. With a pain-free joint the techniques of choice are graded exercise using buoyancy, altered speed of movement or length of weight arm turbulence and patterns of movement.

Group treatments

Once the inflammatory processes have subsided and the person enters the immediate post-acute phase or is in the chronic phase of the disorder, they can be included in a group situation. In such a group generalized exercises are given, followed by specific individual exercises according to the needs of the individual. The starting positions for the exercises can be variable, either lying, sitting or standing, with the exercises modified according to the position. Selected starting positions will be governed by the patient's physical condition.

General Mobility Programme

A general mobility programme along the following lines could be used and include mobility and strengthening exercises, postural awareness, gait retraining and relaxation techniques.

The person should be encouraged to begin with a suggested maximum of ten repetitions for each exercise gradually increasing the number of repetitions as their tolerance permits, and also to work within the limits of pain. Stretching should be encouraged, but a warning against stressing already compromised tissues should be given.

The exercise programme should have a *warm-up* phase, a *specific exercise* phase and a *cool down* phase. For the more able the warm-up phase of three to four minutes in a depth of water at xiphisternum level may consist of rhythmical walking through the water, in changing directions, with exaggerated arm and trunk movements. For the less able the warming phase may be in a depth of water at xiphisternum level with alternate leg and arm movements in different directions followed by trunk rotations and side flexion movements. The period of time can be set at three to four minutes with 10–15 repetitions of each movement. With the emphasis on gentle rhythmic movement there should be minimal stress on joints and peri-articular structures. The cool down phase can include swimming, walking, relaxed trunk and arm movements at a gradually decreasing rate of activity.

At the end of the warm-up phase, group members are positioned for the specific exercises. For those who are unable to stand for long periods or by virtue of disability, or for those who are fearful of deep water most lower limb exercises can be done in the lying position, but in this instance for ease of description, all exercises will be described as for the standing patient; alternative positions being given where appropriate.

Legs

Starting position: the person stands in the water, preferably in a depth in which buoyancy is neutral. Ideally this means the water should be at the level of the xiphisternum. Some people may need to exercise with the water at waist level where there is a greater degree of gravity acting on the body, providing a feeling of greater security to the nervous or anxious person. If the patient has been taught the skills of mental adjustment and balance restoration such action may be obviated (see p. 17).

Exercises that form the basis of the 'conventional' method, that is buoyancy assisted, neutral or resisted exercise, (Davis and Harrison, 1988) and utilize all movements of the hips, knees and feet may be used. Care must be taken with the application of those exercises that take the legs into adduction, across midline. Smaller joints such as the ankle, are less effectively exercised in the water, as a rule, but movements that are aimed at flexibility of the feet and ankles should not be ignored. Approaching these exercises using the principles of hydrodynamic exercise (Chapter 1) are of value. The warmth of the water, the support and buoyancy producing relaxation allow greater mobility without the stresses of a gravity dominated situation and thus there is merit in including exercises that develop flexibility in the ankle and foot in any programme.

Posture

The posture of some patients suffering from rheumatic disorders is altered and exercises and activities that will improve this altered posture should be included in the programme. Taking patients with a forward flexed posture into deeper water, whilst in the vertical position, will often bring about a more upright stance. Since buoyancy has taken the stress off the weight bearing joints and spine and with the patient's natural desire to keep the face and mouth clear of the water, a more erect posture results. Specific exercises involving the quadriceps, gluteal, abdominal, shoulder retractors and neck muscles are carried out to improve trunk-control along with exercises for the trunk muscles. Whilst these exercises are frequently carried out in standing they may also be performed siting on a chair with the shoulders immersed.

Back mobility

Flexion, extension, lateral flexion and rotation of the trunk can be developed in both the sitting and standing positions. The choice of depth is important as it is inadvisable to allow the head to go under the water when performing forward flexion and lateral flexion. A wide base, in either standing or sitting is important for balance, and this is achieved by having the patient stand with the feet wide apart sideways, or in sitting placing the feet apart and keeping the head forward. Once again depth is important.

Arms and shoulders

These exercises should be carried out in the sitting or standing starting positions with the depth of water at shoulder level. Movements that involve flexion, extension, abduction, adduction, internal and external rotation can be used for the shoulders. All these movements should be carried out as rhythmical swinging actions and various components can be combined. The shoulder girdle may be exercised by movements involving elevation, depression, retraction and protraction.

Hands

There is no specific advantage of doing hand exercises in water other than that the warmth of the water promotes ease of movement, and relaxation and that all joints are thus included in the programme. All movements of the fingers, thumbs and wrists should be included, care being taken not to stress the metacarpophalangeal joints or spread into ulnar deviation.

Thought should be given to exercises that combine a variety of movements in functional patterns. As the movements considered above have been discussed in relation to group work the physiotherapist is not able to carry out Bad Ragaz patterns which require a one-to-one relationship between the patient and the physiotherapist. Yet these patterns incorporate all the movements both anatomical and physiological of joints and muscles. It is possible there is a place for the appropriate timetabling of group sessions to permit individual work with the patients so that more functional patterns involving all joints of the limbs may be utilized (Reid Campion, 1988).

Neck

Neck movements can be made more effective if techniques carried out on a one-to-one basis are used (see pp. 27–28).

To exercise the neck effectively in water is not easy and requiring the patient to be immersed as fully as possible if the patient's neck is to benefit from the warmth of the water a stable position is essential. This may be achieved if the patient is seated securely on a chair or leaning with the back against the wall, the hips, knees and ankles flexed and the feet placed flat on the floor of the pool, well forward of the body and wide apart. The movements of the neck and head of flexion, extension, side flexion and rotation can be performed, but should not be continued if they cause dizziness or nausea. The physiotherapist should be aware of any bony destruction or instability of the cervical spin and proceed with care.

Functional activities

Functional activities can be promoted in water although differences occur to similar activities on land due to buoyancy. The advantages of the support of water, warmth, weight relief and relaxation encourage and motivate the patient to carry out such activities early thus facilitating their use on land. There is a psychological benefit for the patient in being able to achieve movement and perform activities with greater ease than without the benefits of water. Functional activities include:

- sitting to standing
- standing balance on both legs or either leg
- walking forwards, sideways and backwards
- stepping up and down.

Balance is a vital factor in all functional activities and can be increased in a variety of ways. Both static and dynamic balance may be developed by means of hydrodynamic exercise (p. 26) and with the use of turbulence.

Relaxation

Relaxation is brought about by the support and warmth of the water. It is important that apart from the body the neck, shoulders and arms are relaxed. Rhythmical, relaxed sweeping movements of the arms may also involve the trunk but the emphasis is on the release of tension from the neck and shoulder areas. Increased range of motion can be achieved by encouraging the patient to gently 'stretch' into the movements.

Swimming

Patients who have swum in the past may find swimming a useful means of activity, maintaining mobility, fitness and providing social and psychological benefits. Care should be taken in choosing the stroke or strokes for a patient.

Generally floating on the back and sculling is suitable for most patients and this can be extended to a backstroke action. Sidestroke may prove suitable for some patients, but careful consideration must be given to the selection of breaststroke. Cervical, thoracic and lumbar extension may be compounded in breaststroke and the kick into abduction and extension with rotation of the lower limbs may stress the lumbar spine, hip and knee joints. Swimming skills should be taught to the non-swimmer and adaptations made for physical disabilities and limited mobility. General teaching techniques for strokes (Elkington, 1978) and modifications for disabilities (Reid Campion, 1985) may be employed.

SAFETY AND CARE IN THE HANDLING OF THE RHEUMATOID ARTHRITIS PATIENT

The handling and holding of the rheumatoid arthritis patient is of utmost importance to prevent an increase of pain and damage to compromised and painful joints, soft tissues and osteoporotic bones. When lifting or transferring patients from a chair to the hoist, commode, chair or wheelchair, care should be exercised by holding the patient around the chest wall, using the length of the lifter's arms. The lift should *not* be done by lifting under the shoulders, *nor* by grasping the patient's forearms or wrists (as is commonly done with a through arm lift). Support for the legs should be given under the *thighs* and the *lower legs*.

When employing a standing transfer to the hoist, support from the helper should be given around the body, not grasping the upper arm and dragging on the shoulder(s). Support, whilst lifting the legs, should be given under the thighs and lower legs, so there is no strain on the knee joints. As the patient is lowered on the hoist into the water, the physiotherapist, already standing in the water, should place one hand or arm over the legs to prevent the legs floating up due to buoyancy and also to reassure the patient against the sensation of floating away (see fig. 6.1).

When transferring from the hoist, the patient should be requested to keep their arms folded over their chest to prevent pulling on the patient's shoulders and to prevent the patient grasping around the physiotherapist's neck due to panic, or should an emergency arise whereby the physiotherapist would be needed to move quickly and unhindered. The person should be held firmly around the body and close to the physiotherapist with one arm whilst the physiotherapist's other arm supports under the person's thighs. In this manner, the patient feels secure, can be floated across the pool and positioned appropriately into the standing position or either lying, sitting or standing.

If the patient is supported on a plinth, a restraining band may be secured firmly across the hips and abdomen and a neck support placed beneath the cervical spine. In this position the patient can perform arm, leg and trunk side flexion and rotation exercises. If the patient is seated on a chair, a restraining band may be placed over the hips and abdomen and firmly secured. Many patients, if fearful of tipping over, may need the chair to be placed near the wall of the pool. The patient should be instructed to keep their head forward in order to maintain the upright position.

When standing a severely disabled rheumatoid arthritis patient from the supine float position, often the most comfortable and secure method is for the physiotherapist to have one arm around the body supporting behind the shoulders and in some cases the head as well. The other hand and forearm is placed over the front of the patient's thighs. An upward pressure is applied to the body by the arm supporting behind the shoulders at the same time a downward pressure is applied by the arm across the front of the thighs, equally, until the patient is brought to an upright position with the feet on the bottom of the pool. As the legs go down and the centre of

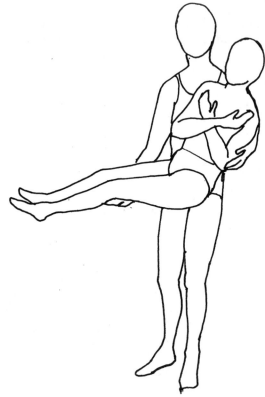

Fig. 6.1

equilibrium is established, the arm pushing on the legs should be moved to support the body at waist level or on the rib cage. If possible, the patient should be encouraged to tuck the chin in, bringing the head forward at the beginning of the movement; blowing out strongly will further facilitate this action of the head. This method is used successfully and comfortably for most persons with severely limiting rheumatoid arthritis, who are unable to employ the self-righting method of forward rotation used in the Halliwick method (see fig. 6.2).

To walk the severely disabled or fragile patient, the physiotherapist should stand in front of and facing the patient. The physiotherapist's hands should hold and support preferably at waist level or over the lower rib cage. The patient rests their hands and forearms

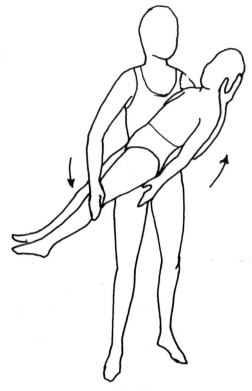

Fig. 6.2

forearms along the physiotherapist's forearms, distributing the
weight away from the patient's wrists. In this way facial expression
can be observed and gait can be analysed and corrected. A feeling of
security is provided by the support to the trunk and the patient can
bear weight along the forearms without stressing the wrists and
hands.

To transfer the patient onto the hoist, the reverse procedure to
that of transferring into the pool is used. The physiotherapist
should maintain a restraining hold over the front of the legs until
the hoist is raised from the water. If the neck or back are painful
during the transfer, either into or out of the water, consideration
should be given to providing some support by means of rubber
cushions or neck supports. The patient's comfort is of paramount
importance at all times.

Safety Points

Whilst acknowledging the following points are applicable to all patients the author feels it is essential to emphasize them here in relation to the handling of the rheumatoid arthritis patients. A number of points for safety should be remembered. Buoyancy can over-ride equilibrium of the elderly or debilitated patient, so the righting position should be taught (Martin, 1981; Campion, 1983; Reid Campion, 1985).

Poor eyesight, hearing, fear of the water, reflection of the light on the water, turbulence of the water, noise and echo and lack of understanding of body mechanisms can all lead to confusion and stress for many patients, particularly the elderly, frail or severely disabled. Awareness of the over-enthusiastic person must also be considered. This person, on finding himself in a warm and welcoming medium, can lean to over-activity and a subsequent increase of pain and swelling.

The use of ladders and steep stairs for entry or exit into or out of the pool should be discouraged because of the degree of stress placed on affected joints and weakened muscle groups. Entry and exit for the rheumatoid arthritis person should, in preference, be either by hoist, ramp or wide shallow steps and the method of entry is determined by the degree of disability.

New or nervous patients should be oriented to the pool beforehand, either by explanation, or better still, by a tour of the pool site itself. Mental adjustment and balance restoration skills should also be taught (p. 16).

Pool therapy is tiring, thus following a pool session the patient should shower, be adequately rested and warmly wrapped or clothed. A minimum of 15 minutes and preferably up to 45 minutes should be allowed for heart rate, respiration, blood pressure and skin temperature to return to normal. Patients should take some fluid refreshment to replace body fluid loss (Atkinson and Harrison, 1981; Golland, 1981).

Treatment times are variable according to the patient's tolerance. For some severely disabled patients, 5 minutes may be enough, initially whilst others may work for 20 minutes without adverse side effects. A full exercise programme can be achieved in 20 minutes, but many patients, particularly the fitter osteo-arthritic or ankylosing spondylitic, will tolerate a session of up to 45 minutes or more, but no longer than one hour, depending on the water temperature and the severity of the condition and exercise. Patients with respiratory or cardio-vascular problems generally tolerate only a short period of treatment (Harrison, 1980; Atkinson and Harrison, 1981; Golland, 1981 (Skinner and Thomson, 1983)).

DEGENERATIVE ARTHRITIS

The conditions treated under this heading include osteoarthrosis, a common disorder of central and peripheral diarthrodeal joints; disc degeneration, also a common disorder frequently co-existing with osteoarthrosis; and osteoporosis of the spine. The most common signs and symptoms will be pain, muscle spasm and weakness and loss of range of motion.

Treatment of Osteoarthrosis (OA)

The aims of treatment for OA are similar to those for inflammatory arthritis. They include relief of pain; relief of muscle spasm; strengthening of the muscles around the affected joints; increased range of motion of the affected joints; improved walking pattern where the lower limbs are involved and encouraging and teaching swimming skills.

Techniques

The techniques employed include relaxation, mobilizations using hold–relax methods, strengthening using Bad Ragaz patterns, stabilizations and repeated contractions, re-education in walking and the teaching or promotion of swimming skills (Elkington, 1978; Reid Campion, 1985). In most cases of OA especially where the hips and knees are involved there is an associated low level of general fitness and mobility and one aim of treatment should be to improve strength and mobility of the trunk muscles.

'Free' exercise programme for osteoarthritis

As in all exercise programmes there should be a 'warm-up' session. Warm-up activities should take place in an appropriate depth which means that the water should be at xiphisternum level if the patient is safe exercising at that level. Such activities include exercises for the legs, arms and trunk using the 'conventional' method (Davis and Harrison, 1988) and walking in various directions.

Specific exercises for the affected joints would aim to increase the range of motion in all directions of movement at the joint(s) as well as strengthening the muscles around those joint(s). Progression for strengthening can be achieved by attaching floats to the limbs, or increasing the speed of the exercises. The starting positions for the exercises may include standing, sitting, kneeling and support lying both supine and prone. Special consideration of the osteoarthritic spine, back pain and the osteoporotic spine is provided on p. 131.

Walking

The physiotherapist should observe and correct abnormal patterns of gait. Instruction should begin with a discussion on posture, correction of the patient's posture, analysis and demonstration of the normal walking pattern. The walking pattern on land is not the same as that for walking in the water. Different muscle work is involved due to the effect of buoyancy assisting and resisting movements of the lower limbs and to the effects of turbulence around the body (Reid Campion, 1985; Davis and Harrison, 1988). The patterns of movement for walking which demand balance and coordination described in Chapter 1 may be used. These patterns can be modified, either by the physiotherapist instructing the patient to make for example, smaller ranges of movement, smaller steps depending on the mobility and ability of the patient to balance.

Functional activities

Functional activities particularly those involving the lower limbs are most important for the osteoarthritic patient. These would follow similar activities to those already described (p. 135) but emphasis would be placed on ascending and descending the 'stairs'; the latter being stools of various heights. It is important that the physiotherapist ensures correct functioning especially of the quadriceps muscle using buoyancy assisted (concentric) and buoyancy resisted (eccentric) exercises.

Swimming

All swimming strokes may be utilized but the physiotherapist must assess the patient's mobility, at the same time being aware of the movements involved in all the strokes, and must ensure that no movement aggravates any joints and produces pain.

Osteoarthrosis Spine, Back Pain, Osteoporotic Spine

The back conditions most commonly seen amongst the arthritic disorders result from inflammatory and degenerative conditions, for example spondylosis, spondylolisthesis and osteoporosis. Many patients may be overweight, underfit, immobile and have poor posture, all brought about by pain, muscle spasm and weakness. The whole person needs treating, but care must be taken to treat within the point of aggravation of signs and symptoms.

Aims of treatment

The aims of treatment are to relieve pain and muscle spasm; to mobilize, specifically the spine and generally the whole body; to strengthen the abdominal, back extensor, hip and leg muscles; to correct the posture; to improve general fitness; to create body awareness and to educate in and promote back care. Selection of appropriate exercises will depend on the findings of the individual's assessment.

It is important that extra care is given with the choice of exercises for the osteoporotic spine, particularly with extension and rotation exercises. The emphasis should be on gentle mobility exercises with a gradual progression of strengthening exercises. The leg muscles must be exercised as well as the trunk muscles.

The physical properties of water can allow for the gradual progression of exercise in terms of weight relief since the effects of buoyancy increase with depth. In the horizontal position, exercises can be totally non-weight bearing, whilst in the vertical position weight bearing can be gradually increased by decreasing the depth of water.

Techniques

The techniques of choice would be those for relaxation which as stated earlier (p. 131, 136) maybe commenced in flotation. Mobilization can be obtained through the Bad Ragaz patterns specifically designed for the trunk.

Free exercise programme

Free exercises should be performed within the point of aggravation of any symptoms. The exercise routine commences with a general warm-up session which would include relaxed neck and shoulder exercises so that tension in those areas is relieved. The starting positions may be that of standing, sitting or lying. Whichever position is used the patient should be immersed as deeply as possible.

Free exercises involve movements of the upper and lower limbs, the trunk, head and neck. When neck exercises are performed specifically for cervical mobility they follow the movements and guidelines provided on p. 27. The usual progressions of exercise such as, increasing the speed, the range of motion and the repetitions can be utilized.

Isometric exercises can be included for muscle strengthening, for example standing with the back against the wall, pressing the arms against the wall, holding then relaxing. Posture correction should be included by getting the patient to practise tightening the quadriceps, the gluteals and the abdominals at the same time as retracting the scapulae and elongating the cervical spine by stretching the crown of the head towards the ceiling.

Balance, posture and walking skills must be maintained. Balance control not only involves control in standing on both feet but includes the ability to counteract the effects of buoyancy and turbulence. Ways in which balance can be maintained and improved are given in Chapter 1. In all these exercises an upright posture is desirable and the patient requires careful instruction about posture correction and maintenance. Walking should be practised in all directions with the resistance being varied by increasing the speed of motion and therefore, the turbulence around the moving body.

Swimming

Patients are encouraged to swim using any stroke which is comfortable; generally the stroke of preference is back stroke to prevent hyperextension. For the osteoporotic patient, backstroke again would be the choice as it involves most work for the posterior shoulder girdle muscles and thoracic spine movements. Breaststroke may be used, but only if there is no discomfort due to hyperextension of the spine, especially the cervical spine.

SPONDYLOARTHROPATHIES

The conditions grouped under this heading are also known under the heading of 'sero-negative spondarthritis' and include such conditions as ankylosing spondylitis, psoriatic arthritis, Reiter's disease, ulcerative colitis or Crohn's disease (Moll, 1980). A similar exercise routine can be applied for all conditions. The example used is for ankylosing spondylitis.

Ankylosing Spondylitis

Ankylosing spondylitis is a sero-negative inflammatory arthropathy affecting mainly the axial skeleton, but it may involve some peripheral joints such as the hips, shoulders, knees or feet. It is characterized in the early stages by low back pain, stiffness and impaired chest mobility; in the later stages by permanent stiffness, intermittent episodes of pain, loss of range of motion of the spine and possibly of the hips and shoulders, the latter often due to soft tissue contractures.

Aims of treatment

In the early or *acute stages* of the condition where pain is the predominant feature, the aims of treatment are to relieve pain and muscle spasm; to increase respiratory expansion, function and vital capacity; to maintain mobility of the spine, hips and shoulders; to create body awareness and to establish postural habits.

In the later stages of the condition when pain and muscle spasm are reduced and on into the *chronic stage* of the disorder, the aims of treatment are as stated for the early stage, but attention is paid also to increasing muscle strength to counteract deformities; to improving mobility and to teaching or improving swimming ability.

It is of interest to note that the Chartered Physiotherapists Policy Statement (*Physiotherapy*, January 1979) gives as a contra-indication to hydrotherapy, chest conditions where the vital capacity is below 1500 cc; a statement which would exempt some people with ankylosing spondylitis and a low vital capacity, from participating in hydrotherapy. However, Harrison (1981) disputes this figure and it has been the experience of this author that a low vital capacity and/or restricted chest mobility in the person with ankylosing spondylitis is no reason to preclude the person from an active hydrotherapy programme.

Technique

In the early or acute stages individual treatment is preferable, particularly if pain and muscle spasm are the predominant features. On a one-to-one basis it is easier to gain relaxation of muscle spasm by having the person supported in floats with the physiotherapist passively moving their body from side to side in large movements, inducing relaxation. Once relaxation is achieved the person is encouraged to assist the movement actively

Breathing exercises can also be introduced with the person actively trying to expand the rib cage laterally or by the physiotherapist assisting by passively moving the trunk into side flexion to gain unilateral chest expansion. Mobilization of the trunk and limbs can also follow once relaxation has been achieved using the Bad Ragaz patterns of movement involving the trunk and upper and lower limbs (Bolton, 1971; Boyle, 1981). Swimming can be introduced at the early stage with the person choosing the stroke they find most comfortable and which does not aggravate the pain or muscle spasm. In the case of non or poor swimmers, water safety should be taught using the Halliwick principles (Martin, 1981; Campion, 1983; Reid Campion, 1985).

Free exercise programme

Free exercises for the patient with ankylosing spondylitis can be divided into early and later rehabilitation programmes.

From the beginning, the programmes are active ones which place great emphasis on chest mobility, neck movements, posture, trunk, hip and shoulder mobility. Relaxation can be practised either by floating with supports or freely using large sweeping movements of the limbs and trunk. As with any exercise programme a 'warm-up' session is important. Emphasis should be on lateral costal movement rather than diaphragmatic breathing. Some patients may find the pressure of the water on the chest wall uncomfortable, in which case the exercises can be carried out in supine lying on a plinth with part of the chest clear of the water. As the patient is able to tolerate the pressure so the starting position is changed to standing. Trunk movements may be combined with the breathing patterns to increase mobility and flexibility in the spine.

Neck exercises can be carried out in the 'more usual' manner in a free exercise programme but it is suggested that a more effective method of working the neck muscles is for the physiotherapist to work individually with the patient using both the flexed position and rolling techniques previously provided (p. 27). Good posture is vital for the patient with ankylosing spondylitis and in treatment this should be emphasized. Arm movements, with the importance of scapulae retraction and shoulder extension being stressed, assist in good postural control. Breaststroke arm action for example can achieve this type of movement.

Trunk mobility is developed through the 'conventional' trunk exercises emphasizing the extreme ranges of movement with over pressure to increase the range. Combining arm and trunk actions assists trunk mobility. Trunk movements may be carried out lying on a plinth in various positions, and when leg movements are incorporated they prove helpful in mobilizing the trunk and hip joints.

All exercises should be governed by the amount of pain and modifications to an exercise should be determined by individual needs. In the later stages of rehabilitation the exercise programme is expanded and the work load added to by increasing the speed which ensures there is greater turbulence effect and therefore, requires more effort and a greater range of movement is developed.

Flotation equipment may be used for some exercises to increase the work load. For example, an exercise for the trunk and shoulders could be progressed by the use of a flotation ring. With the arms in the 'reach' position and grasping the ring with the hands the patient swings the arms from side to side at the same time rotating the trunk. At the end of the range of movement to each side the patient pauses and attempts to push the ring under the water at the same time extending the trunk.

The various arm movements for the swimming strokes of overarm, breaststroke and backstroke can be incorporated in the programme and combined with body movements. The speed of the arm movement can be varied and breath control included by encouraging the patient in breathing techniques used for individual swimming strokes (Elkington, 1978; Reid Campion, 1985).

Stretching techniques (in a group)

A number of techniques can be used effectively to stretch tightened structures particularly of the hips, hamstring muscles, trunk and shoulders by the use of floats and buoyancy assistance. The method of contract–relax then employs passive stretching. Adequate fixation is necessary to localize the movement. The stretches should be done three times to maximize the effect before changing to the opposite side or limb (Barefoot—Lecture Notes 1988).

The physiotherapist's imagination and ingenuity can devise a wide variety of exercises and activities for these patients in a free programme. Such programmes should be interesting, and varied regularly as these patients will require a considerable amount of treatment over the years. Provided the aims of treatment are incorporated there are no limits to the activities that can be developed.

Hydrodynamic exercises may be used to strengthen muscles, particularly those of the trunk, and to increase the range of motion. These may be incorporated in free programmes provided they have been taught carefully and frequent checks are made to observe that the patient is carrying out the exercises correctly.

Swimming

All the swimming strokes can be attempted with modification according to the needs of the individual and the problems associated with stiffness. It may be necessary for some people to have a neck ring and hip float to enable them to perform back stroke. Others may be unable to perform breaststroke due to spinal rigidity. Underwater swimming can be included, not only to improve breath control, but as a competitive incentive. Some swimmers employ the use of a snorkel to overcome the problems due to stiffness. As there is some medical concern over breath holding in under-water swimming, controlled blowing out should be encouraged, whereby the air is gradually expelled from the lungs. (Strauss 1982; Reid Campion, 1985).

Posture check

Before leaving the water, a posture check can be carried out as a reminder to maintain an upright stance and correct head position. Standing with the feet slightly apart, the knees are braced into extension by tightening the quadriceps, the gluteals and abdominals are tightened to control pelvic tilt (an integral part of posture correction and awareness), the shoulders are drawn back by adducting the scapulae and the head position corrected by extension and retraction of the lower cervical spine attempting to glide the neck back at the cervical, thoracic level. This movement is followed by cervical elongation by stretching upwards from the crown of the head.

FIBROSITIS

Fibrositis, a regional pain syndrome, is a common cause of musculoskeletal pain and disability. Other terms commonly used for this condition include fibromyalgia, fibromyositis and myofascial pain syndrome (Yunus, 1983). Fibrositis is an important cause of rheumatic symptoms and in an Australian study it was suggested that approximately 10% of rheumatology referrals had the fibrositis syndrome (Moran *et al.*, 1984). Various studies have been conducted to establish definable clinical features, although the pathophysiology of the syndrome is poorly understood (Yunus *et al.*, 1981; Campbell *et al.*, 1983; Wolfe, 1986).

Clinical symptoms

The symptoms of fibrositis include chronic aches, pains and stiffness in various areas of the body, including joints, muscles, ligaments, tendon insertions, subcutaneous tissues and bony prominences (Zilko, 1986). All patients have multiple areas of local increased tenderness called tender or trigger points (Smythe, 1985). Other major symptoms include disturbed sleep, morning stiffness and fatigue. Management is variable, but should generally include reassurance, education, restoration of good sleep pattern relaxation etc. relaxation training and advice about exercise, both a specific programme and general fitness (Moran *et al.*, 1982; Zilko, 1986).

Treatment

Hydrotherapy is beneficial for persons with fibrositis, particularly if the syndrome is chronic and well-established. With the body weight being supported by buoyancy and with the water temperature relaxing tense muscles, range of movement and muscle extensibility can be increased. Initially gentle muscle stretching and mobility exercises are used, and then, as pain decreases, strengthening exercises can be included, particularly for the trunk musculature.

The following programme for the fibrositis patient forms the basis of the exercise regimen of a research programme being conducted by the author and colleagues. All the exercises are carried out in a level of water at the xiphoid process. Exceptions are made when the shoulders are being exercised; the water should then cover the shoulders; the neck should be immersed as far as possible when it is being moved. This ensures that the parts being exercised benefit from the warmth, buoyancy and support of the water. For the patient with fibrositis it would be difficult to perform some of the exercises on land because pain would be increased working against gravity. In particular exercises 2,4, and 5 would be extremely likely to produce pain on land, and may be used more readily in water.

1. Arm circling, forward, back and around, with the elbow flexed (Fig. 6.3).
2. Alternate hip–knee flexion towards chest (Fig. 6.4).
3. Hip abduction with the patient lying on a plinth, in floats or standing (Fig. 6.5).

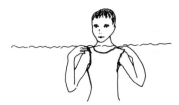

Fig. 6.3 Arm circling

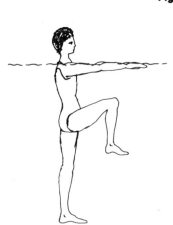

Fig. 6.4 Hip–knee flexion

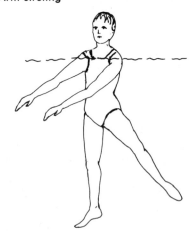

Fig. 6.5 Abduction of hip in standing

4. Horizontal abduction/ adduction of the arms. The arms are at shoulder level and may be supported on floats (Figs. 6.6 and 6.7).
5. Shoulder protraction/retraction, with arms floating straight out in front and moving alternately (Fig. 6.8).
6. Upper trunk rotation, swinging head, shoulders and arms around, with feet and hips kept still (Fig. 6.9).
7. Shoulder girdle circling.
8. Cervical rotation and side flexion (Figs. 6.10 and 6.11).

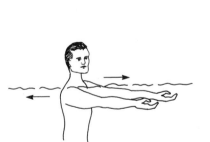

Fig. 6.6 Abduction of the arms

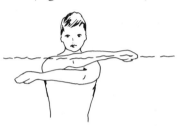

Fig. 6.7 Adduction of the arms

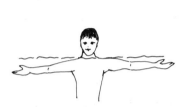

Fig. 6.8 Shoulder retraction/protraction

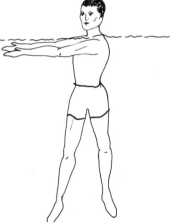

Fig. 6.9 Upper trunk rotation

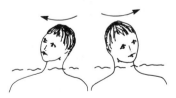

Fig. 6.10 Cervical rotation

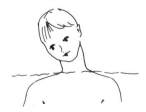

Fig. 6.11 Cervical side of flexion

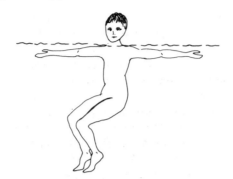

Fig. 6.12 Lumbar rotation

9. Lumbar rotation, done against the wall with hips and knees flexed and arms stabilized along the wall (Fig. 6.12).

Walking in the water is also useful, both sideways, encouraging lateral flexion, and forwards, where posture correction should be included.

Hydrodynamic exercises may be added to assist in strengthening trunk musculature by asking the patient to maintain the static posture as the body shape in the water changes. Turbulence may be used behind the patient to increase the difficulty of the exercise. This can be done by the physiotherapist rapidly crossing the arms from side to side directly behind the patient.

As pain becomes less of a problem, then muscle strengthening can be enhanced by using some Bad Ragaz techniques. A number of the trunk patterns are applicable, and in particular the following:

1. Lower trunk lateral flexion
2. Lower trunk flexion/rotation
3. Cervical and thoracic extension

Generally, the patient with fibrositis should continue a hydrotherapy programme regularly to maintain good mobility and to relieve pain from tense muscles. Once the patient has been examined carefully and a specific hydrotherapy programme has been given and evaluated over a number of sessions by the physiotherapist, then often the programme can be continued long term by the patient without supervision. Patients with mild symptoms may well progress to swimming as a form of general fitness training.

REFERENCES

Atkinson G.P., Harrison R.A. (1981). Implications of the health and safety at workout in relation to hydrotherapy departments.

Barefoot J. (1988). Unpublished lecture notes. *Physiotherapy*, 67(9), 263–265.

Barefoot J. (1988). Unpublished lecture notes.

Bolton E., (1971). A technique of resistive exercise adapted for a small pool. *Physiotherapy*, 57(10), 481–482.

Bolton E., Goodwin D. (1974). *An Introduction to Pool Exercises*, (4th edn.). London: Churchill Livingstone.

Boyle A.M. (1981). The Bad Ragaz method. *Physiotherapy*, 67(9), 265–268.

Campbell, S.M., Clark S., Tindall E.A. *et al.* (1983). Clinical characteristics of fibrositis 1. A 'blinded' controlled study of symptoms and tender points. *Arthritis and Rheumatism*, 26(7), 817–824.

Campion M. (1983). Water activity based on the Halliwick method. In (Skinner A.T., Thomson A.M. eds.) *Duffield's Exercise in Water*, London, Baillière Tindall.

Davis B.C., (1967). A technique of re-education in the treatment pool. *Physiotherapy*, 63(2), 57–59.

Davis B.C. (1971). A technique of resistive exercise in the treatment pool. *Physiotherapy*, 57(10), 480–481.

Davis B.C., Harrison R.A. (1988). *Hydrotherapy in Practice*, Edinburgh: Churchill Livingstone.

Elkington H.J. (1978). *Swimming: A Handbook for Teachers.* Cambridge: Cambridge University Press.

Golland, A. (1981). Basic hydrotherapy. *Physiotherapy*, 67(9), 258–262.

Harrison R.A. (1980). Hydrotherapy in rheumatic conditions. In *Physiotherapy in Rheumatology*, (Hyde, S. ed.), Oxford: Blackwell Scientific Publications.

Harrison R.A. (1981). Tolerance of pool therapy by ankylosing spondylitis patients with low vital capacities. *Physiotherapy*, 67(10), 296–297.

Martin J. (1981). The Halliwick method. *Physiotherapy*, 67(10), 288–291.

Moll J.M.H. (1980). *Ankylosing Spondylitis*, Edinburgh: Churchill Livingstone.

Moran H., Barraclough D., Littlejohn G. *et al.* (1984). Referral patterns in suburban private rheumatology practices. *Australia and New Zealand Journal of Medicine*, 14(3) (suppl. 1), 367.

Orwoll E.S., Ferar J.L., Oriatt S.K. (1987). The effect of swimming exercise and bone mineral content *Abstracted Clin. Res.* **35(1)**, 194A.

Reid Campion M. (1985). *Hydrotherapy in Paediatrics*, Oxford: Heinemann Medical.

Reid Campion M. (1988). Unpublished lecture.

Smythe H.A. (1985). Fibrositis and other diffuse mucoloskeletal syndromes. In (Kelley *et al.* eds.) *Textbook of Rheumatology*, 2nd edn. p. 481. Philadelphia: W.B. Saunders Company.

Strauss R.H. (1982). Concerns in underwater sports, *Pediatric Clinics of North America*, **29(6)**, 1431.

Wolfe F. (1986). The clinical syndrome of fibrositis. *American Journal of Medicine* **81** (suppl 3A), 7–14.

Yunus M.B. (1983). Fibromyalgia syndrome: a need for uniform classification. *Journal of Rheumatology*, **10**, 841.

Yunus M.B., Masi, A.T., Calabro J.J. *et al.* (1981). Primary fibromyalgia (fibrositis): clinical study of 50 patients with matched normal controls. *Seminars in Arthritis and Rheumatism* **11**, 151.

Zilko P.J. (1986). Fibrositis syndrome. Diagnosis and management. *Patient Management*, 10(4): 35–44.

ADDITIONAL READING

Berson D., Ray S. (1979). *Painfree Arthritis (Exercises in Water)*. Boston: G. K. Hull.

Cadogan, D.R. (1971). Handling the Handicapped. *Physiotherapy*, **57,10**, 467–470.

Dick, W.C. (1972). *An Introduction to Clinical Rheumatology*, Edinburgh and London: Churchill Livingstone.

Elkington H.J. (1971). The effective use of the pool. *Physiotherapy*, **57(10)**, 452–460.

Fries J.F. (1979). *Arthritis: A Comprehensive Guide*, Massachusetts: Addison-Wesley Publishing Co.

Gardiner M.D. (1963). *Principles of Exercise Therapy*, (3rd edn.), London: G. Bell and Sons.

Harris S.J. (1971). Bathside management, pool hygiene and resuscitation. *Physiotherapy*, **57(10)**, 471–475.

Harrison R.A. (1980). A quantitative approach to strengthening exercises in the hydrotherapy pool. *Physiotherapy*, **66**, No. 2. p. 60.

Harrison R., Bulstrode S. (1987). Percentage weight bearing during partial immersion in the hydrotherapy pool. *Physiotherapy Practice*, **3**, 60–63.

Hart F.D. (1981). *Overcoming Arthritis*, Sydney: Methuen Australia Pty. Ltd.

Jagger M., Smood D. (1984). Hydrotherapy by physiotherapists in a community health clinic. *Australian Family Physician*, **13(12)**, 878–881.

Jetter J., Kadlec N. (1985). *The Arthritis Book of Water Exercise*. London: Granada Publishing Co.

Kacavas J., Morrison D., Thurley M. (1977). The use of aqua therapy with geriatric patients. *American Corrective Therapy Journal*, **31(2)**, 52–59.

Reed, B., Rose, M. (1985) *Water Workout*. Melbourne: MacMillan Sun Books.

Roth A. (1975). Therapeutic Water Exercise: A treatment modality in orthopaedic management. *Journal of Western Pacific Orthopaedic Association*, **XII(1)**, 15–20.

Scott J.T. (1980). *Arthritis and Rheumatism*. Oxford: Oxford University Press.

Trussell E.C. (1971) Swimming for the disabled. *Physiotherapy*, **57(10)**, 461–466.

Tinsley L.M. (1983). Ankylosing spondylitis programme, *Australian Physiotherapy Newsletter (W.A.)*, 9–12.

Wynn Parry C.B., Deary J. (1980). Physical measures in rehabilitation. In *Ankylosing Spondylitis*. (Moll J.M.H. ed.) Edinburgh: Churchill Livingstone.

Williams L. (1987). Get wet, get moving. *Western Australian Arthritis & Rheumatism Foundation Newsletter*, No. 73.

Hydrotherapy in Orthopaedics

The field of orthopaedics is wide and varied with many conditions and degrees of severity from trauma to elective surgery. Due to the diversity, it is impossible to describe hydrotherapy programmes for every conceivable orthopaedic problem. The ensuing chapter deals with many of the orthopaedic conditions and surgery seen at the Royal Perth Rehabilitation Hospital, Perth, Western Australia. It by no means covers every condition but should give the reader an insight into the hydrotherapy treatment of musculoskeletal problems.

Signs and Symptoms

The signs and symptoms encountered in the orthopaedic patient may include: pain, muscle spasm, oedema, loss of balance, muscle weakness, loss of joint range caused by pain, stiffness or a combination of the two and an altered gait pattern.

- The benefits gained by immersion in warm water affect all of the above signs and symptoms.
- *Pain* will be reduced by the all-round warmth which decreases the sensitivity of nerve endings. Water supports the body and therefore, the injured part, which together with the reduction of gravity and weight on the injured part, should result in a reduction of pain.
- *Muscle spasm*—if the pain is decreased, it follows that relaxation of muscles takes place. Warmth aids relaxation and decreases muscle spasm.
- *Oedema* will be decreased as the pressure acting on a part increases with increasing depth, thus aiding venous return, if the part is exercised as deep as possible.
- *Loss of balance* is aided by the upward thrust acting on a body equal to the fluid it displaces (Archimedes principle).
- Water supports the body, the effect of gravity is easily reduced, thus gait training may be accomplished without the use of walking aids.

- *Muscle weakness* is affected by the warmth of the water, which increases the circulation to the muscles and therefore, increases their overall function. A fine progression of exercise can be obtained more easily in water than in the gravity dominant situation on land.
- *Loss of joint range*—as the pain decreases, the joint range of motion should increase. Stiffness may be decreased by joint mobilizations, the fine progression of resistive exercise and specialized techniques such as hold–relax.
- *Altered gait pattern* may be observed in many orthopaedic conditions, requiring the use of a walking aid, which alters the normal gait pattern dramatically. In water, the walking aid can be dispensed with and a more normal pattern be adopted, although this will not be as normal as a gait pattern on land, as buoyancy assists and resists different parts of the movement incurred in walking. This may also be finely progressed by using varying depths of water during treatment.

Many conditions encountered will have different levels of weight bearing on land, i.e. non-weight bearing, partial weight bearing and light weight bearing. The hydrotherapy pool is regularly used for initial weight bearing, using different depths. The weight passing through the patient's lower limbs can be progressed in a controlled manner.

Harrison and Bulstrode (1987) researched the percentage weight bearing at different depths related to the anatomical landmarks on male and female subjects. Thus, by referring to Table 7.1 and the patient's weight, the physiotherapist can accurately gauge the amount of weight bearing at any depth.

Pease and Flentje (1976) found that a pre-ambulation programme of 15 min twice a day, commencing in water at the axillary level and graduating to shallower levels as the patient's condition improves, is extremely beneficial in lower extremity injuries, e.g. knee ligament tears, hamstring strains and ankle sprains.

Table 7.1 Percentage weight bearing when immersed in water

Level	Female	Male
C7	8%	8%
Xiphisternum	28%	35%
ASIS	47%	54%

from Harrison and Bulstrode (1987)

Assessment and Record Keeping

It is of extreme importance to perform an initial assessment prior to the patient entering the pool (see p. 14). Goniometry is important when treating joint problems; it is often overlooked due to lack of time or difficulty in reading under water. Joint ranges should be recorded before entry, in the water, after the exercise in the water and again out of the pool. In this way, an accurate record can be kept and used to demonstrate if a specific exercise is helpful or detrimental.

Classwork—Yes or No?

In many hydrotherapy pools, nowadays, the number of patients requiring treatment can be daunting. There is a fine line between trying to satisfy the masses and being unsafe. Safety is of utmost importance, the physiotherapist must be in reach at all times of his patients. Many elderly people are referred for hydrotherapy, some may never have been in a pool in their lives and so are very unsure, or a patient's body shape may have changed since last being immersed in water. The physiotherapist must be aware of these factors and spend time on each individual's needs.

Bad Ragaz techniques which are carried out on a one-to-one basis are not therefore, suitable for large classes. However, it is possible to timetable such patterns into programmes for small classes. The individual needs of each patient should be catered for in any programme. To some extent this can be achieved where the class is formed of patients with similar conditions and performing similar exercises, and time spent during the session by the physiotherapist working with each participant.

Swimming Strokes

Swimming is an excellent exercise for weak muscles and the cardiovascular system, but each patient must be assessed thoroughly to ascertain the appropriateness of each type of stroke.

Suture Lines

Many orthopaedic patients will have wounds of some kind, either

Table 7.2

Movement Produced	Type of Stroke
Hip flexion and extension	• frog kick (breaststroke) • scissor kick (side stroke) • flutter kick (crawl stroke)
Hip abduction and adduction	• frog kick (breaststroke) • scissor kick (side stroke)
Hip internal and external rotation	• back stroke
Knee flexion and extension	• side stroke • frog kick • crawl and back stroke
Ankle plantarflexion	• all strokes
Ankle dorsiflexion	• some work is performed prior to kick phase of strokes
Shoulder	• varying amounts of shoulder movements occur in all strokes, therefore a combination of strokes may be needed
Elbow flexion and extension	• is involved in most strokes
Forearm and wrist	• all strokes
Pronation and supination	• sculling
Wrist flexion and extension	• sculling
Hand	• paddle for all strokes

from an accident or from surgery. A contra-indication of hydrotherapy is open wounds, therefore common sense and a close liaison with the doctor is essential.

Skinner and Thomson (1983) state that hydrotherapy may commence as soon as sutures are removed, usually 10–14 days postoperatively. However, some patients may start as early as five days provided the necessary precautions are observed, i.e. there is not any leakage from the wound, any gaping of the wound and no infection present and the wound is in good condition. A plastic dressing can be sprayed over the sutures to make it waterproof.

Exercise Progression

Haralsun (1986) states that exercises may be either buoyancy assisted, buoyancy supported or buoyancy resisted.

1. Buoyancy assists the limb when moved passively to the

surface of the water. The effect can be increased by adding a float or lengthening the lever arm.

2.   Buoyancy supports the limb when the part is moved horizontally across the water's surface. The resistance can be increased as speed is increased, causing increasing impedance. Colson and Collison (1983) state that the degree of resistance offered by water depends on the surface area of the part moved and the rate of movement. An increase in speed causes an increase in resistance as a turbulent effect is seen, a negative pressure behind the direction of movement.

3.   Buoyancy resists movement when the part is moved downward from the surface. Resistance may be increased by increasing the speed lengthening the lever arm or adding floats.

With Bad Ragaz techniques, the patient is in float support lying, therefore, with buoyancy supporting, progression may be achieved by the speed of movement, thus increasing bow wave or drag effect and the number of repetitions.

Bad Ragaz techniques may be performed isometrically or isotonically, either unilaterally or bilaterally, whilst hydrodynamic exercises may be employed symmetrically or asymmetrically (see Chapter 1). Other specialized techniques available are hold–relax, stabilizations and repeated contractions. These specialized techniques are extremely beneficial to muscle strengthening and increasing joint range. Skinner and Thomson (1983) state that when the range of a joint is limited by muscle spasm, hold–relax techniques are employed. The starting position and joint stabilization is important and buoyancy is used to assist the joint into the required range. A starting position in deeper water is used and the physiotherapist uses her body and hands to stabilize unaffected joints and to avoid trick movements. The use of stabilizations for co-contraction and hold–relax techniques are beneficial once a thorough assessment is undertaken with special reference to muscle spasm. Stabilization may be used in the water to produce co-contraction at the joint. Repeated contractions are used to increase the endurance of a muscle and are valuable in re-educating a muscle group by using turbulence or turbulence and buoyancy. The above techniques may be used for all the following conditions:

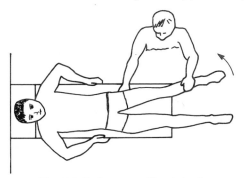

Fig. 7.1 To increase hip abduction

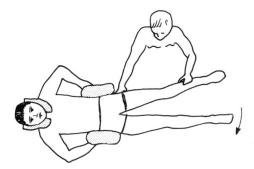

Fig. 7.2 Right leg is working, i.e. abducting

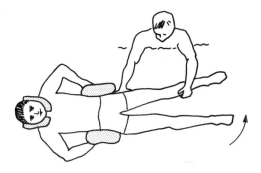

Fig. 7.3 Right leg is working, i.e. adducting

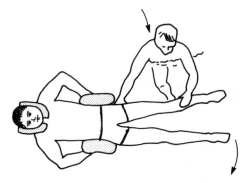

Fig. 7.4 Repeated contractions right hip abductors

ORTHOPAEDIC CONDITIONS

The orthopaedic conditions discussed will be divided into specific areas of the body.

Pelvis

Triple pelvic osteotomy

Triple pelvic osteotomy is performed mainly for those persons with congenital hip dislocation, where the acetabulum is shallow and malformed. In later life this may lead to extreme pain and alteration of function.

Four weeks of Hamilton Russell traction is commonly used post-operatively, therefore, once the patient commences mobilization he has lost much muscle strength and balance. A period of non-weight bearing ambulation using crutches follows.

Hydrotherapy may commence immediately after the traction has been removed. Due to the long period of immobilization muscle atrophy, postural hypotension, joint stiffness and a reduction in cardio-vascular fitness would be evident. Hydrotherapy is extremely beneficial in initally allowing the patient to relax in the warmth thus providing easier movement of the upper and lower limbs. The pressure exerted by the water aids reduction of lower limb oedema. Once movement and confidence are gained, gait re-education may be commenced in neck deep water and a graduated exercise programme for the hips and knees is followed.

Fractures of the pubic rami

Fractures of the pubic rami may be unilateral or bilateral and involve the superior or inferior pubic rami. The treatment is conservative and the patient is allowed to mobilize within the limits of pain. Due to the extreme pain, gait re-education on land is difficult, but is more readily carried out in water. The aims of hydrotherapy in this condition are to strengthen the muscles on the affected side, to increase hip range of motion and to re-educate balance and gait.

Entry into the pool—patients with triple pelvic osteotomy or fractures of the pubic rami should be hoisted into the pool initially because of their pain. In the case of fracture pelvic osteotomy, the patient is not able to weight bear through the affected limb, but once the patient begins crutch walking, a ramp may be used. In the case of the fractured pubic rami patient, pain is the determining factor as to when a ramp may be used for entry to the water.

Exercises—hydrotherapy treatment of the above conditions may include: hip abduction, adduction, flexion and extension exercises which are performed in standing. Progression of these exercises is achieved by adding resistance, e.g. side walking or by utilizing a Bad Ragaz pattern of isotonic unilateral hip abduction. Gait re-education is important at this stage and is best commenced at xiphisternum level in the pool and progressed as improvement is seen, to a shallower depth. Bad Ragaz techniques are very versatile and can be useful to the practised physiotherapist and may be modified to the individual patient.

Hip Joint

Fractured neck of femur

This usually occurs in the elderly and the main complication of this condition is avascular necrosis of the head of the femur. Surgical intervention is common and may take the form of pin and plate, hemiarthroplasty or total hip arthroplasty.

These elderly patients may be apprehensive regarding treatment in the hydrotherapy pool. They should be reassured by explanations that they do not have to swim and that the exercises will be carried out in standing or supported lying. Further adjustment to water can take place once in the water by applying the principles of mental adjustment and balance restoration.

The greatest benefit of hydrotherapy in these cases is in gait re-education. Pain is a predominant factor when ambulating on land. The reduction of weight in water decreases the pain which in turn allows greater movement and a more appropriate gait pattern. The movement of hip abduction is performed in standing or supine plinth lying, whilst hip flexion and circumduction are carried out in standing ensuring that the patient is stable. Ambulation, both forwards and sideways should initially take place with the water at xiphisternum depth progressing to the shallower end of the pool.

Aims of treatment—the aims of treatment are to strengthen the muscles around the hip, maintain or increase hip range of motion, gait training and general maintenance exercises.

Entry into pool—the method of entry to the pool depends on the level of rehabilitation. If the patient has not ambulated independently on land, the hoist would be used until a satisfactory level of independence is reached.

Exercises—the main danger in total hip arthroplasty is dislocation and less so in hemiarthroplasy. Therefore, as a general rule, the affected limb should not be adducted past midline or flexed past 90° and both external and internal rotation be limited. Fixation by the pin and plate method is strong and no limits of movement are set, unlike the two previous conditions.

Total hip replacement

Two types of total hip arthroplasty are currently used. The first is cemented and the second uncemented. Many different post-operative regimens may be used, but generally the cemented hip is allowed to partial weight bear immediately and the uncemented hip may be either partially weight bearing or be completely non-weight bearing.

This dictates the depth in which the patient is treated when standing. For non-weight bearing patients, a water level at C7 would be appropriate, whereas the partial weight bearing patient may stand at a lower depth which initially does not go below the xiphisternum level.

Entry into pool—the method of entry to the pool for the patient who is permitted to partially weight bear is a ramp. For the non-weight bearing patient, the hoist is used initially. However, if the patient has strong upper limbs the ramp may be used.

Exercise—hydrotherapy is especially beneficial in regaining hip movement, muscle strength, gait re-education and allows for a graduated exercise programme. This programme includes hip abduction in standing or supine plinth lying, hip flexion in standing which must not exceed 30 degrees, hip extension, knee flexion and extension in standing. Bad Ragaz patterns for abduction using both isometric and isotonic muscle work may be included in the programme. If other Bad Ragaz patterns are used care must be taken in regard to the rotary components as rotation is contra-indicated in certain instances. This applies to 'conventional' type exercises also.

Dangers and precautions—the main danger is dislocation in total hip arthroplasty. The physiotherapist must know which incisional approach was employed during surgery as each approach has different dangers. An anterior incision means that the movement of extension and external rotation presents a danger. A postero-lateral incision means that adduction, flexion and internal rotation are movements posing a threat, whilst a posterior approach means that flexion forms a threat. The physiotherapist must also be aware of whether the patient is non-weight bearing and treat him accordingly. As a general rule strong resistance is avoided in the total hip arthroplasty, though the resistance of the water may be used.

Girdlestone arthroplasty

The operation for girdlestone arthoplasty is performed after a failed total hip replacement, recurrent infection or if it is the only operation possible. Traction usually follows surgery. When mobilization is allowed, one difficulty that exists is that of shortening. This is overcome by a build-up to the shoe worn on the affected side.

Aims—the aims of treatment are to strengthen the muscles around the hip and to re-educate gait; movement is not usually a problem.

Entry into pool—the preferred method of entry to the pool with girdlestone arthroplasty is the hoist.

Exercises—hydrotherapy in this case is beneficial in that it allows the patient a sense of freedom from the difficulties of early ambulation on land. It allows them to be in a vertical position again while being supported. Hip exercises on the affected side may be carried out as for total hip replacements, within the patient's limits of pain. Resisted exercises to the unaffected limb are an important part of the programme, Bad Ragaz techniques being an excellent choice of treatment.

Dangers and precautions—there are not any real dangers with the hip itself, although the physiotherapist must exercise the patient within the limits of pain. It is difficult to re-educate a gait pattern in the pool with this procedure due to the limb shortening and depending on the pool used; the floor may be sloping, further emphasizing the problem of unequal length. It is useful to use a boot with the appropriate build-up in the pool.

Slipped Upper Femoral Epiphysis

Occurs mainly in young males and is corrected at surgery by pinning the head of the femur. Occasionally, prophylactic pinning is performed on the unaffected hip.

Aims—the aims of treatment are to strengthen the muscles around the hip, to maintain or increase hip range motion.

Entry into the pool—the method of entry to the pool is the hoist initially, and as patient is able he may enter via the ramp

Exercises—hydrotherapy is commenced at an early stage (approximately one week postoperatively). Pain is at this time usually the major complaint, restricting movement and ambulation. Once in the pool, movement becomes easier and gentle non-forceful exercises may commence e.g. hip abduction in standing or supine support plinth lying, hip flexion in standing, knee flexion and extension with a resistive component and ambulation in water at the C7 level.

Dangers and precautions—patients with slipped upper femoral epiphysis are required to be non-weight bearing and it is safer not to take the hip to its extremes of range and to put any undue stress on the site of pinning. If disrupted, avascular necrosis to the head of the femur may result.

Fractured shaft of femur

A very common fracture seen in orthopaedic wards around the world. Treatment may be conservative with bed rest and traction, or it may be treated surgically by an intramedullary nail (a closed type of fixation) or the fracture may be plated (an open fixation). The severity of the fracture determines the time at which mobilization may commence. At the time of mobilization, the patient may be allowed to weight bear or he may have to remain non-weight bearing.

Aims—the aims of treatment are to strengthen the muscles around the hip and knee, to increase knee range of motion and to re-educate gait.

Entry into the pool—the method of entry to the pool is the hoist initially for non-weight bearing patients and those with bilateral fractures. A ramp may be used for those who are partially weight bearing.

Exercise—after long periods of immobilization lower limb joints become stiff and respond well to hydrotherapy. In addition gait re-education which is easier in water than on land may be commenced early. The treatment programme could include the whole gambit of hip and knee exercises from buoyancy assisted through to buoyancy resisted movements. Bad Ragaz patterns and eventually gentle swimming activity, taking into account the severity of the condition, the age and fixation of the fracture.

Dangers and precautions—at the time of the fracture, there may be extensive quadriceps muscle damage, more so with a compound fracture. During the recuperation period, the damaged muscles heal in a shortened position and tethering may be seen. It is important to remember this when treating such a patient and not to apply excessive force into flexion. Quadriceps atrophy is pronounced after immobilization. This tends to alter the patient's centre of balance resulting in a rotation force which makes it difficult for the patient particularly when floating supine. The patient needs to be taught how to control the rotational effects and achieve balance in any position.

Knee Joint

Total knee replacement

Several types of total knee replacement prostheses are used, most tending to be uncemented as opposed to the earlier cemented and constrained prosthesis. After surgery the patients commence partial weight bearing ambulation from one to three days. Flexion exercises may sometimes commence immediately. Depending on the condition of the suture line, hydrotherapy can be commenced seven to ten days post surgery. Post-operatively, a problem can be a quadriceps lag and the patient is sometimes required to wear an extension splint until the lag is reduced to zero. The patient is not required to wear this splint in the pool.

Patients who have had a total knee replacement find considerable difficulty flexing and extending the knee on dry land. The hydrotherapy pool is an excellent treatment medium in which to overcome this problem. The patients are aware of the decrease in pain once in the water and therefore, tend to gain range of movement and are better able to ambulate.

Aims—the aims of hydrotherapy treatment are to increase the range of motion of the knee, to strengthen the quadriceps and hamstring muscles and to re-educate gait.

Entry into pool—the method of entry to the pool can be by the ramp, unless some other problem exists, e.g. severe rheumatoid arthritis affecting the joints, where the hoist would be used.

Exercise—knee flexion may be carried out when standing as buoyancy will assist the movement. To ensure pure buoyancy assisted knee flexion, the physiotherapist must instruct the patient to keep the knees together and the thighs in line. Such instructions prevent hip flexion occurring at the same time as flexion of the knee takes place. In the sitting position knee flexion is resisted by buoyancy when the movement takes place from an extended position. Floats may be added to increase the work load. Bicycle pedalling, hold–relax techniques, ambulating at various depths in all directions and Bad Ragaz patterns, both isometric and isotonic are useful. Extension of the knee can be encouraged by 'conventional' method exercises, and is involved in Bad Ragaz patterns.

Dangers and precautions—there are not any real dangers with regard to movement, only from open suture lines and the fact that the physiotherapist should not force the knee into flexion.

Knee reconstruction (soft tissue)

This operation is performed for knee instability, resulting from ruptures of either anterior cruciate ligament, post cruciate ligament or the collateral ligaments. Many of these patients are young sports persons. After surgery, rehabilitation time is quite lengthy; the knees are placed in a support, which is angled at between 30–60° to allow the healing of soft tissues to occur in a shortened position, therefore increasing stability later on. The knee is kept in this splint for approximately six weeks and ambulation is non-weight bearing. After this time, an exercise programme is commenced and hydrotherapy may begin.

Aims—the aims of treatment are to strengthen muscles affecting the knee, to increase knee range of motion, to re-educate gait and to improve cardio-vascular function.

Entry into the pool—the method of entry to the pool is the ramp.

Exercise—at the end of six weeks of immobilization the affected lower limb has lost a lot of muscle bulk and the range of motion is limited in both flexion and extension. Hydrotherapy is useful in that it allows easier movement, initial light weight bearing ambulation, a graduated exercise programme and with a swimming programme, an increase in cardio-vascular fitness.

Exercises should be gentle at first, without heavy resistance incorporating both flexion and extension components e.g. flexion in standing (buoyancy assists) and progressing on to sitting flexion from an extended position (buoyancy resists) to sitting with a float attached to the ankle, starting from an extended position to Bad Ragaz patterns of isometric and isotonic flexion to swimming (side stroke and frog kick). Extension of the knee would use the opposite of the above with the swimming strokes being the crawl and backstroke. The aim with knee reconstructions is to gain the range of motion without the joint being forced.

Dangers and precautions—the affected knee should not be forced into extension.

Supracondylar fracture, tibial plateau fracture and fractured patella

Each of these fractures communicates with the joint surface and thus an effusion is the result which, with immobilization, leads to a stiff knee. There may be different levels of severity, so the commencement time for hydrotherapy depends on this and the method of treating the fracture, either by internal fixation or conservative management. Many of these patients commence ambulation non-weight bearing which is difficult and energy consuming on land but easier and safer in water. It should commence with the water at C7 level and be progressed to shallower depths as more weight bearing is allowed.

Aims—the aims of treatment are to increase knee range of motion, to decrease the quadriceps lag, to strengthen the quadriceps and hamstring muscles and to re-educate gait.

Entry into pool—the method of entry to the pool depends on the level of mobilization. For non-weight bearing patients, the hoist may be used initially and for those who are allowed to weight bear, the ramp may be used.

Exercises—as with knee reconstructions, exercises should begin gently and progress as improvement in range of motion and healing take place. A programme of flexion and extension exercises using buoyancy to assist, support and then resist should be carried out. Isotonic Bad Ragaz patterns that involve flexion and extension of the knee are useful and other patterns, both isometric and isotonic, may be utilized to maintain unaffected joints and muscles.

Dangers and precautions—the severe fractures should not take weight through the affected limb until sound union takes place. A comminuted fracture of the patella may be restricted from flexing the knee. A tibial plateau fracture remains non-weight bearing for six weeks.

Tibial osteotomy

This operation is performed when either the medial or lateral compartment of the knee is taking most of the weight, i.e. in severe valgus or varus deformities. After surgery, the knee is placed in a cylinder of plaster of paris for four to six weeks, after which mobilization is commenced. The patients are allowed to be full weight bearing.

Aims—the aims of treatment are to increase range of motion of the knee, to strengthen quadriceps and hamstring muscles and to re-educate gait.

Entry into pool—the method of entry to the pool is via the ramp.

Exercises—knee flexion is the most restricted movement and needs considerable attention. Conventional method exercises in all positions so that buoyancy assists, supports and resists are useful. Floats may be added to progress muscle work and increase the range of motion; hold–relax techniques and Bad Ragaz patterns, especially those of flexion, adduction, lateral rotation, knee flexion, dorsiflexion and inversion and the bilateral isotonic/isometric pattern (Boyle, 1981). The hydrotherapy treatment of these patients can be more vigorous than the preceding conditions and can be progressed at a faster rate.

Dangers and precautions—the knee should not be forced into flexion.

Ankle Joint

Fractured tibia and fibula

This is a common fracture which can affect both the knee and ankle joints. The method of treatment may be conservative in a full cylinder plaster of paris for 8–12 weeks, or operative fixation where the fracture is plated and a plaster worn for appoximately six weeks. A problem in operative fixation is wound breakdown due to thinness of soft tissue covering the tibia. When the plaster cast is removed, the knee and ankle may be stiff and the quadriceps, hamstrings and ankle muscles will be weak. Ambulation is usually partially weight bearing. Where the fracture involves two joints both should be treated. Fractures near or involving the ankle joint benefit from gait training in water. The use of walking aids necessary on land are discarded for the hydrotherapy sessions and a fine progression of graduated weight bearing may be achieved by changing the patient's position to a shallower depth. Exercising in deep water helps to reduce oedema (Pascal's Law). Standing on the affected leg and balancing against turbulence deliberately produced by the physiotherapist can aid the rehabilitation of movement and proprioception at the ankle.

Aims—the aims of hydrotherapy treatment are to increase knee and ankle range of motion, to strengthen muscles affecting the knee and ankle and to re-educate gait.

Entry into pool—the method of entry to the pool, if non-weight bearing, is the hoist and later the ramp, when sufficiently mobile and if partial weight bearing.

Exercises—the Bad Ragaz pattern for dorsiflexion and plantarflexion, and other patterns that involve ankle movements combined with knee and hip movements can be used successfully. Hydrodynamic exercises in the sitting position (p. 26) may prove beneficial, especially an exercise which produces dorsiflexion when the hips are dropped downwards towards the heels and water adjusts the body's balance. Particular attention should be paid to each phase of the gait pattern during ambulation. Swimming may be used later in the rehabilitation programme; some dorsiflexion is involved in the preparation of the kick phase of strokes and can be augmented by the addition of flippers. Plantarflexion takes place in all strokes.

Dangers and precautions—the physiotherapist should be aware of the strength of fixation and degree of union of the fracture.

Tibialis posterior transfer

This is an operative treatment for foot drop, i.e. transferring the tibialis posterior tendon for use as a dorsiflexor of the ankle. After surgery, a below knee plaster cylinder is applied for approximately six weeks. During this time the patient is allowed to partially weight bear. After removal of plaster the new action of the muscle has to be trained and ankle stiffness reduced.

Entry into the pool—the method of entry to the pool initially is the hoist, then when ambulating safely, the ramp.

Exercise—this may be achieved with the use of Bad Ragaz techniques. In this case, treatment in water, due to buoyancy, is partial weight bearing, thus exerting less force on the ankle than on land. The warmth of the water also leads to a decrease in pain, and proprioception may be developed by the use of turbulence.

Dangers and precautions—gait may be quite unsteady at the beginning due to poor muscle control of ankle movement and a decrease in the ankle proprioception.

Shoulder Joint

Fractured neck of humerus

This is a common fracture in elderly patients and often treated conservatively in a sling. A problem that exists with this injury is pain and large amounts of oedema and bruising. The patient is reluctant to move the limb, which in turn may become stiff, the muscles atrophy and loss of function results. Pendular exercises are begun at once and active abduction encouraged within the limits of pain. Exercises in the pool may also begin at once, initially in a sitting position and progressing to standing ambulation and eventually the arm movements of swimming strokes when ambulating. The physiotherapist should be aware when treating shoulder problems that trick movements are common.

Aims—the aims of treatment are to increase range of motion of the shoulder joint and to strengthen muscles around the shoulder.

Entry into the pool—the method of entry to the pool is via the ramp.

Exercises—these patients find great relief from hydrotherapy. The warmth of the water aids relaxation and buoyancy supports the arm thus giving the patient confidence and allowing movement of the shoulder more easily than on land.

The hydrotherapeutic programme would include the movements of flexion, extension, abduction and adduction in sitting. A weighted chair on which the patient sits at a depth of water that covers the shoulders is used. The patient should be instructed to keep the head forward so that the feet stay down on the floor of the pool and balance is not placed at risk. If there is any doubt in regard to the patient's ability to maintain the position a strap which is attached to the chair should be placed around the patient for security.

To progress the movements of flexion, extension, abduction and adduction a paddle may be introduced to increase resistance. Once fracture healing is well under way Bad Ragaz techniques can prove extremely useful as they have a rotatory component. Swimming is also beneficial for gaining range of movement, muscle strength and cardio-vascular fitness but the age of the patient and previous swimming ability must be considered. A combination of strokes may be used to develop whatever mobility is possible.

Dangers and precautions—movement should not be forced, and rotatory movements avoided initially, and introduced cautiously.

Arthroplasty

There can be two types, either a hemiarthroplasty with the humeral head being replaced or a total arthroplasty with both the glenoid and humeral head being replaced. A strict post-operative regimen at the Royal Perth Rehabilitation Hospital is followed with these patients and commencement of hydrotherapy and movements should be considered accordingly. This regimen is derived from the Neer shoulder arthroplasty post-operative programme, and is as follows:

Table 7.3

Days postoperatively	Exercises
6	● Pendulum exercises commenced
8	● assisted extension
	● reciprocal pulleys into flexion
10	● assisted internal and external rotation
	● isometric internal and external rotation
	● isometric extension
	● isometric abduction
12	● active anterior elevation
	● resisted extension
21	● full range active movement into elevation, internal rotation, external rotation and extension.

Hydrotherapy usually commences about 12–14 days post-operatively when the sutures have been removed. The above regimen is adapted to the water with care being taken until the 21st day post-operatively when full range active movements are permitted. On land most movements, up to three weeks are either active assisted or isometric. In water the patient can undertake different movements with buoyancy assisting, thus fulfilling the criteria of only assisted movements.

Shaft of humerus

A common fracture of younger patients. The fracture is immobilized for six to eight weeks, after which time it is removed and exercises begin. Stiffness of the elbow is more likely than in the shoulder, as shoulder movements can be performed gently during the period of immobilization.

Aims—the aims of treatment are to increase shoulder and elbow range of motion and to strengthen muscles around elbow and shoulder.

Entry into the pool—the method of entry to the pool is via the ramp.

Dangers and precautions—movement should not be forced.

Elbow Joint

Fractures around the elbow require immobilization in a plaster cylinder for up to six weeks; then mobilization may commence. Joint range is gained without many problems and muscle strength of biceps and triceps is important for the stability of the joint. Elbow arthroplasty, although not a common procedure, may be performed in cases of extreme injury or rheumatoid arthritis. Fractures of the radius and ulna are a common injury and are treated conservatively with immobilization in a plaster cylinder for six weeks. In these cases, the wrist may become stiff and muscles of the forearm atrophy.

Aims—the aims of treatment are to increase elbow range of motion and to increase the muscle strength of the elbow.

Exercises—elbow exercises are limited and therefore, Bad Ragaz arm patterns are useful as they combine shoulder and elbow movements. When performing 'conventional' method exercises floats or paddles may be used to aid abduction of the shoulder.

Swimming using a combination of strokes is beneficial. Movements of the shoulder are more involved in swimming, but elbow movements are less affected although breaststroke offers a greater range of motion than other strokes.

Dangers and precautions—movement into flexion or extension should not be forced.

Hydrotherapy is of enormous value in the treatment of orthopaedic conditions. Its advantages far outweigh the disadvantages, allowing early mobilization in a medium that aids relaxation, supports the body and allows a fine progression of exercise.

REFERENCES

Boyle A. M. (1981). The Bad Ragaz ring method, *Physiotherapy*, **67**, 9.

Colson J. H. C., Clllison, F. W. (1983). *Progressive Exercise Therapy*, 4th edn., p. 56, Bristol: Wright.

Harrison R., Bulstrode S. (1987). Percentage weight bearing during partial immersion in the hydrotherapy pool. *Physiotherapy Practice*, **3**: pp. 60–63.

Haralsun K. M. (1986). Therapeutic pool programs, *Clinical Management*, **5(2)**, 10–12.

Pease R. L., Flentje W. (1976). Rehabilitation through underwater exercise. *Physician and Sportsmedicine*, **4(10)**, 143.

Skinner A. T., Thomson A. M. (1983). *Duffield's Exercise in Water*, 3rd edn., London: Ballière Tindall.

Diana HOPPER

Hydrotherapy for Sports Injuries

Hydrotherapy has been used in sports medicine for centuries, generally in the form of whirlpool baths and natural hot springs. During the 1940s, underwater exercises became more popularized in the treatment of polio and severely wounded soldiers. Even today with the increased number of swimming pools available, exercises in water for pleasure, fitness and/or rehabilitation is a relatively new phenomenon. In Australia one of the latest exercise fads is aqua-aerobics. These exercise classes are conducted in water and are set to the beat of music. With pressure from elite and professional injured athletes, the swimming pool is becoming very important in rehabilitation and fitness maintenance of the athlete.

The treatment of sports injuries using hydrotherapy is far more extensive than just having a non-specific swim or a paddle in the water! The injured athlete can utilize the pool and train both anaerobically and aerobically so that specific energy systems related to a particular sport can be maintained. In addition, specific rehabilitation programmes enable the athlete to train during the early stages of the injury, otherwise rest or non-weight bearing exercises would be recommended. In recent times, hydrotherapy is one of the most underutilized and underestimated methods of treatment in sports injuries. With more exposure and an increased success rate in the rehabilitation of sports injuries, hydrotherapy must become the integrated treatment regimen of the future.

When an athlete is injured, he wants to get better yesterday! Therefore, there is enormous pressure on the physiotherapist to rehabilitate the athlete as soon as possible. Traditional treatment of sports injuries during the acute phase include ice, elevation, compression, gentle exercises, strapping, inferential therapy and ultrasound. Treatment regimens change during the sub-acute and chronic phases of rehabilitation. These regimens become more exercise orientated with some assistance from electrophysical agents such as high voltage stimulation and laser therapy. On certain occasions and for specific conditions, traditional physiotherapy treatment programmes are limited, especially for non-weight bearing rehabilitation, for example, the overuse lower limb injuries. These types of athletic injuries can now be treated using the swimming pool. Here, exercises can be designed specifically to suit their problem and also can maintain aerobic and anaerobic fitness specific to their sport. The principles of both physiotherapy and hydrotherapy treatments for the sports injuries described in this chapter would apply to most, if not all, sports injuries. Minor modifications related to the condition may need to be made. This chapter proposes to focus on how hydrotherapy can enhance the treatment of sports injuries and is divided into the following sub-headings:

1. The classification of injuries
2. Common conditions treated by hydrotherapy
3. Principles of rehabilitation
4. Organization of a hydrotherapy treatment programme
5. Running in water

1 The Classification of Injuries

- Extrinsic—is an injury that is due to an external force.
- Intrinsic—is an injury that is due an internal derangement.
- Overuse—is a repetition strain beyond the body's limitation.
- Unaccustomed use—is a repetition strain caused by unfamiliar external factors.

2 Common Conditions Treated by Hydrotherapy

Sporting injuries are usually treated by the traditional land base treatment regimens such as strapping, exercises, electrophysical agents and other ergogenic aids. Water has the added advantage of buoyancy which can relieve the stresses of weight bearing on joints. When the injury is characterized by pain and muscle spasm, relief of these signs and symptoms can be obtained by immersion in warm water. In the sub-acute phase, bruising and swelling can be affected by the warmth of the water. This increases the circulation and facilitates the dispersion of the waste products. Furthermore, swelling can be aided by the pressure of water on the affected area, particularly if the part is exercised in water which is as deep as possible. This principle supports Pascal's law of pressure which increases with the depth of water. If the athlete suffers from limitations of movement, temporary muscle weakness, incoordination, decreased balance and altered gait patterns, then activities in the pool can be very helpful.

The healing process is well documented in the literature. However, Evan's (1980) article succinctly illustrates the different stages of inflammation and repair. In the early stages of inflammation, hydrotherapy would *not* be recommended but in the sub-acute and chronic phase of healing, hydrotherapy would be recommended as an excellent treatment regimen which will be further discussed.

SKELETAL PROBLEMS

Stress fractures

Stress fractures present quite frequently in sports injury clinics. It is a condition that affects bones rather than soft tissues, and is common among athletes especially long distance runners. Roy and Irvine (1983) indicate that factors clearly associated with stress fractures are muscle forces acting across the bone and the impact repetitive mechanical stress on the microtrabecular structure of the bone. Although almost any bone in the body can be affected, Fitch (1979) states that the most likely sites are the femur, tibia, fibula, calcaneus, navicular and metatarsal shafts. Roy and Irvine also include other sites such as the par interarticularis of the lumbar spine, rib and humerus fractures in sports related to gymnastics; weight lifting; tennis and throwing events.

Aetiology

Athletes who train over long distances on hard surfaces and who increase their training workload by more than 10% per week place undue continuous and repetitive strain on their lower limb. Long distance runners are especially prone to this injury. Besides continuous repetitive overload and muscle fatigue, athletes often present with problems related to poor biomechanical running technique and incorrect lower limb malalignment (e.g. excessive pronation of the foot).

Signs and symptoms

The athlete complains initially of pain during activity which is relieved by rest from weight bearing activities. In the next stage the pain continues for hours and frequently becomes worse at night. The athlete is advised to cease long distance running and full weight bearing activities until the fracture site has healed.

Indications for hydrotherapy

Hydrotherapy is an excellent alternative to endurance training. The athlete can maintain aerobic fitness by swimming training in the pool and also by running in deep water supported by a buoyancy aid. As the fracture site heals, the athlete can then progress by running in water partially supported. Specific exercises to correct muscle imbalance problems can also be performed in conjunction with swimming and running in water so that the athlete can maintain optimum fitness and specific training related to the site of the stress fracture.

Specific exercises of the 'conventional' method would be used for the joints below and above the injury site. Exercises would be buoyancy assisted, neutral and resisted and progressed in the usual manner such as altering the weight arm, increasing the number of floats, repetitions and speed. Bad Ragaz patterns would form part of the rehabilitation programme; the patterns employed would again depend on the site of the stress fracture. If a lower limb stress fracture is present, the athlete's unaffected limb should also receive attention. Where the tibia and fibula are concerned any accompanying swelling indicates the need to exercise the part in as deep water as possible (Pascal's law). Initially, 'conventional' method exercises would be carried out at a buoyancy dominant water level, but as the condition improved the athlete would exercise at decreasing buoyancy levels and finally in a gravity dominated situation. In addition to these exercises the use of turbulence suitably placed in front, behind, and to either side of the athlete who is standing on the affected leg in a water level (to the level of the xiphisternum) may be used. At first, the turbulence would be applied gently by the physiotherapist and it would be steadily increased to disturb the athlete's balance. Finally, the physiotherapist would move around the athlete in different directions, thereby creating greater turbulence. The athlete is required to use all the balance mechanisms to maintain the erect position which produces similar unstable effects of the land based wobbleboard.

KNEE PROBLEMS

Ligamentous Knee Injuries

Knee injuries are potentially more severe than any other joint in the body because of its anatomical complexity and importance in gait and movement. The main anatomical structures at risk are the collateral ligaments, menisci and the anterior cruciate ligament (ACL). These structures are particularly valgus force placed on the leg with the knee in flexion and external rotation. The most common ligamentous injuries occur on the medial aspect of the knee sometimes involving the medial meniscus, the medial collateral ligament and the ACL.

If all three structures are involved then the injury is considered serious and is known as the 'O'Donoghue Triad'. Some examples of sports that may be predisposed to these injuries are: different codes of football; netball; skiing and breaststroke swimmers. Counsilman (1968) reports that few of his swimmers develop painful knees and he attributes this to correct execution of the whip kick. Stulberg *et al.* (1980) also supports these findings. In contrast, Kennedy and Hawkins (1974) consider that even with correct technique, the elite breaststroke swimmer is vulnerable to knee injury because of the severity and repetitive stress of the whip kick.

Aetiology

Rovere and Nichols (1985) and Vizsolyi *et al.* (1987) found that knee pain is positively correlated with age, increasing years of competition and specific training characteristics. There is also general agreement that knee pain is located medially and that it is related to the extension or thrust phase of the whip kick. Stulberg *et al.* (1980) report that the fault in style is basically due to excessive hip abduction. Rovere and Nichols (1985) support this view but relate the cause of the abduction fault to limited hip internal rotation. In contrast, Vizsolyi *et al.* (1987) criticize Stulberg's argument of the kick being too narrow as the 'narrow kick' reduces forward propulsion. Adequate outward rotation of the feet is necessary for an efficient thrust, and if not provided at the hips will result in increased valgus and rotary knee stress during subsequent circumduction. Kennedy and Hawkins (1974) found that knee pain occurs during the extension phase of the kick and is possibly related to the increasing tension in the medial collateral ligament from external rotatory and valgus forces.

During most athletic activities such as contact sports (e.g. codes of football, hockey, basketball, netball, etc.) and non contact sports (e.g. fencing, field athletics, skiing, gymnastics) the knee is placed under abnormal stress. Depending upon the nature of this stress, the knee is considered to be in a vulnerable position. Petersen and Renstrom (1986) describe the mechanism of the most common injuries.

1. An impact injury which hits the knee from the lateral side or hits the forefoot from the medial side;
2. An impact injury which hits the knee joint from the medial side or hits the forefoot from the lateral side;
3. An impact injury which results in hyperextension or hyperflexion of the knee joint;
4. A twisting impact without body contact.

Signs and symptoms

The immediate presentation of a knee injury is crucial in the diagnosis. If the knee swells within six hours then the injury is deemed to be serious (Noyes *et al.*, 1980). A haemarthrosis presentation is also considered serious. Often the chronic knee will be limited in movement because of the 'boggy' swelling which needs to be shifted to improve the range of movement. Muscle strength around the knee joint is necessary for knee control and stability. Frequently, the quadriceps muscle atrophies after an injury and Spencer *et al.* (1984) consider this to be largely due to a reflex inhibition. Factors contributing to this inhibition may be related to pain, ligament stretching, capsular compression, joint movement and irritation of the injury (Spencer *et al.*, 1984).

Indications for hydrotherapy

Sub-acute phase—where there is pain, swelling, loss of function, hydrotherapy can be of value. Gentle exercises of the 'conventional' type for the joints below and above the knee would be included in the programme, whilst more vigorous activities would be encouraged for the unaffected limb.

Knee movements would be encouraged within the pain limitations, but owing to the warmth of the water and support pain would be relieved allowing a greater range of movement to occur. If Bad Ragaz techniques are employed, care must be taken not to allow the freedom of movement in the water to increase the range of movement such as to aggravate the injury; this can be prevented by the use of proximal holds in which greater control is exercised both by the athlete and the physiotherapist. Bad Ragaz leg patterns in which the knee is kept straight can be effective in strengthening the quadriceps muscle. The rotatory component of some patterns needs to be watched and modified if pain is manifested. Isometric work can be achieved by using the leg abduction pattern and progressed to isotonic contractions using the single leg abduction and adduction patterns as well as bilateral movements (Skinner and Thomson, 1983). Other patterns using a straight leg with medial and lateral rotation and flexion and extension combination with abduction and adduction can be introduced as the condition improves.

Knee flexion should be introduced gradually. It is essential that this action is isolated from hip flexion when buoyancy assisted knee flexion is required. Exact instructions are given to the athlete as to how to achieve the movement without involving hip flexion, i.e. 'Keep the knees together and the thighs in line'. Swimming in this phase should involve only backstroke and freestyle, thus avoiding the breaststroke whip kick and too much flexion at the knee.

Chronic phase—in this phase, pain, swelling and loss of function may still be present but strength and muscle control are vital. All the above Bad Ragaz patterns that include knee flexion and extension can be introduced and steadily progressed. Swimming would also form part of the programme.

Hydrodynamic exercises may be included in the programme especially as the athlete's range of knee flexion and extension increases. For example, knee extension with dorsiflexion of the foot in the 'sitting' position so that a bubble is caused at the surface by the action of the knee and foot which do not break the surface (p. 30).

SHOULDER PROBLEMS

Shoulder Girdle Injuries

The most common injuries to the shoulder girdle involve the acromioclavicular joint, the sternoclavicular joint, the glenohumeral joint dislocation and rotator cuff impingement syndrome. The glenohumeral joint is a modified ball-and-socket which allows for a greater range of movement and sacrifices stability. This anatomical trade-off is particularly detrimental to the athlete who plays contact sports especially the different codes of football e.g. rugby. Other sports which are often hampered by shoulder problems related to the rotator cuff impingement syndrome are throwing (e.g. baseball pitcher, javelin thrower), serving action (e.g. badminton, tennis) and overarm action (e.g. freestyle, backstroke and butterfly swimming strokes). Whether a competitive or a recreational athlete, pain in the shoulder limits participation. At the elite level, the loss of talent resulting from shoulder injury may significantly reduce the quality and depth of the national team (McMaster, 1986).

Aetiology

Athletes who participate in contact sports often encounter a blow from an external force which results in injuries to the three joints: the acromioclavicular joint; the sternoclavicular joint and the glenohumeral joint. Anterior dislocation of the glenohumeral joint is usually a result of a collision on the playing field, whereas, rotator cuff impingement syndrome is an overuse problem caused by mainly training errors, biochemical faults and muscle imbalance. For instance, in swimming the cocking of the arm in the recovery phase tends to load the lateral undersurface of the acromion and the acromioclavicular joint (Hawkins and Abrahams, 1987).

Shoulder pain is the most common orthopaedic complaint among competitive swimmers, accounting for 37.8% of all injuries treated (Matheson and Gerrard, 1986) and affecting 42–60% of swimmers (Richardson *et al.*, 1980; Penny and Smith, 1986). This repetitive stress of the abduction-forward flexion-internal rotation cycle during training leads to an inflammatory response to micro-trauma that takes place under the coraco-acromial arch. The soft tissue structures implicated in the mechanically induced inflammatory pathology are the supraspinatus tendon, the biceps tendons, the sub-acromial bursa or the shoulder capsule.

Contributory factors include:

- Anatomical impingement of the greater tuberosity, supraspinatus and biceps tendons under the sub-acromial arch (Sarrafian, 1983).
- Hypertrophy of the musculotendinous structures under the acromion (Hawkins and Hobeikea, 1983).

- Impairment of the microvasculature of supraspinatus and the long head of biceps tendon (Rathbun and McNab, 1970).
- Muscle imbalances around the rotator cuff and scapula (Fowler, 1985).
- Poor flexibility round the shoulder joint complex (Griepp, 1985).
- Poor adaptation to training. This can occur when a change of stimulus is too great over a short period or when the recuperative interval between sessions is not sufficient (Fricker *et al.*, 1984).

Signs and symptoms

Usually for the three joints around the shoulder girdle the signs and symptoms become apparent as a specific incident is encountered on the field. This results in pain and loss of normal movement. On the other hand, the rotator cuff impingement syndrome is an overuse problem which occurs with an insidious onset. The pain pattern commences when the athlete initially complains of pain after the activity and as the condition worsens the pain affects performance and finally pain is experienced at rest.

Indications for hydrotherapy

Sub-acute phase—pain, swelling and loss of function are present. The athlete is reluctant to move the arm away from the side. Relaxation may be brought about by supporting the athlete in float lying (Reid Campion, 1985). The physiotherapist walks slowly backwards drawing the person's body through the water gently swaying it from side to side. When the arm is relaxed it will tend to move away from the body due to turbulence which facilitates movement. Once relaxation is gained, buoyancy assisted arm movements are introduced and can be progressed to buoyancy neutral. As the condition improves, further progressions follow and Bad Ragaz isometric arm patterns followed by carefully applied isotonic patterns can be included in the programme. As the joints are potentially painful, proximal holds should be applied in these patterns initially.

Chronic phase—in this phase, the need of strength and muscle control become vital and all the techniques in the sub-acute phases may be extended. The holds for Bad Ragaz patterns could become more distal, particularly if pain reduction has occurred, thus allowing for a greater range of movement and for stronger muscle work. Slow reversals, stabilizations; successive induction and repeated contractions may be used (Skinner and Thomson, 1983). For the rotator cuff impingement syndrome the above treatment would form part of the treatment regimen with emphasis on the correction of training and technical errors.

ANKLE PROBLEMS

Ankle Ligamentous Injuries

Soft tissue injuries to the ankle joint are very common. Roy and Irvin (1980) state that over 80% of all ankle injuries are inversion sprains occurring while the athlete is running straight ahead or cutting. Anatomically, the lateral ligament complex is more vulnerable with 13 separate ligamentous bands compared with the robust ligaments of the deltoid ligament on the medial aspect of the ankle.

Aetiology

The mechanism of injury is important in determining the severity and ligaments involved in the ankle sprain. The anterior talofibular is usually the first ligament implicated in an inversion and plantar sprain. More severe inversion sprains involve the calcaneofibular and the posterior talofibular ligaments. Cutting across the plantar-flexed, inverted foot will create a rotational sprain involving the tibiofibular ligament and interosseous membrane. Eversion sprains are less frequent in occurrence, but when injured the foot often goes into an excessive amount of pronation particularly when moving in the opposite direction.

Signs and symptoms

In most cases ankle injuries present with varying degrees of swelling. This swelling can persist in the sub-acute and the chronic stages and limit the range of movement of the ankle joint. Muscle weakness and poor proprioception in the injured group of muscles can also inhibit rehabilitation.

Indications for hydrotherapy

In the instance of a sprained ankle, treament using the pool has a number of advantages. Pressure according to Pascal's law will help disperse swelling in addition to the increased circulation. Activity should take place in a buoyancy neutral situation initially, that is, with the water level at the xiphisternum or just above. A variety of exercises can be carried out at this level, including standing on the affected leg and balancing against turbulence around the patient by the physiotherapist. A specific treatment regimen would be on similar lines as that described in stress fractures (p. 179).

OVERUSE INJURIES IN THE LEG

Achilles Tendonitis

The Achilles tendon has no synovial sheath which structurally predisposes the athlete to mainly tendonitis problems due to overuse. This injury is very debilitating and can be responsible for the cessation of a successful athletic career. Sports which involve fast repetitive movement (e.g. sprinters, jumpers) and the endurance of long distance runners are predisposed to Achilles tendonitis. Excessive stress on the tendon will lead to inflammation and microtrauma to the soft tissues surrounding the tendon, microscopic tears within the tendon.

Aetiology

Often the onset of Achilles tendonitis is insiduous and gradual. Some of the predisposing factors are related to overtraining, ill fitting shoes, training on roads with a sloping camber and excessive uphill running. All these factors place excessive strain on the tendon. Structural malalignments such as genu valgum and excessive stress on foot pronation also place undue stress on the tendon.

Signs and symptoms

In the acute phase, the athlete complains of pain and swelling along the tendon. Pain is produced during running and climbing stairs rather than walking. Whereas, in the chronic phase, walking is especially difficult at the beginning of the day.

Indications for hydrotherapy

Once the inflammatory response has settled, hydrotherapy is ideal to continue training without placing undue stress on the Achilles tendon. The athlete can maintain aerobic fitness by swimming training in the pool and also by running in deep water supported by buoyancy aids. As the tendonitis improves, the athlete can then progress by running in water partially supported. Specific exercises to correct muscle imbalance problems such as tight gastrocnemius and soleus can also be performed. These would be exercises of the 'conventional' type as well as Bad Ragaz patterns and hydrodynamic exercise (p. 28). These can be performed in conjunction with the swimming and running water programme. During this phase of rehabilitation, the athlete can maintain optimum fitness and specific training related to Achilles tendonitis in the pool.

SPINAL INJURIES

Neck pain is a particular problem which may, at first view, seem not appropriate for treatment in water. However, some specific patterns of movement can be utilized to reproduce cervical flexion, extension, side flexion and rotation. Walking sideways can initiate side flexion or with the athlete held in a ball shape (see Fig. 27) tilting the body sideways can provoke the head righting response thus producing side flexion. In the same position rocking of the body by the physiotherapist forwards and backwards can induce cervical flexion and extension. With the patient lying supine supported by the physiotherapist rolling the body can result in rotation of the head from side to side. This movement can be increased, if the rolling of the body to a flat position again is resisted by the physiotherapist (see p. 28).

Spine

Often athletes strain their backs during training and/or competition especially during contact sports such as football, rugby, soccer and basketball. Mobilization is probably indicated but it is also necessary to treat the strained muscles. Swimming freestyle in a heated pool can relax the muscles and mobilize the joints in a dynamic and functional way. In addition, specific relaxation techniques and gentle rhythmical movements of the upper and lower limbs can also assist in the reduction of pain, swelling and loss of functional movement. Where the pain is very acute simply 'hanging' from the poolside can be beneficial. The athlete would be in deep water so that when 'hanging' the feet are clear of the floor of the pool. The forearms and flexed elbows are placed on the side of the pool and the body is lowered deeper into the water facing the wall of the pool.

The athlete may remain in this position for as long as required to bring relief. There is traction on the structures of the trunk and the warmth of the water also aids pain relief. Relaxation may be obtained as described on p. 43. 'Conventional' methods of exercise may be used but the depth is vital and some actions if carried out in deep water may bring the head very close to the surface of the water or even under the water.

Bad Ragaz arm and leg patterns are introduced as preliminaries to the commencement of the trunk patterns. Whilst performing the arm and leg patterns the athlete will use the trunk musculature to stabilize the body. Leg pain, if present may be reduced by careful application of lower limb patterns. The trunk patterns should begin with the physiotherapist stabilizing the pelvis and the legs and gently moving the person through the water in an arc whilst the athlete holds a static midline position against the turbulence created by the passage of the body through the water in one direction or the other. Further patterns which involve side-flexion, flexion and extension and later rotation may be introduced and progressed as the athlete's condition allows. Hydrodynamic exercises are useful adjuncts to the programme in the later stages of rehabilitation (see p. 28).

3 Principles of Rehabilitation

For an injured athlete to be rehabilitated, details of the sport itself must be understood so that the athlete can be specifically rehabilitated to the demands of the playing position of that sport. To assist with this process of rehabilitation, the physiotherapist can use the following headings as a check list:

- know the player's position
- know the demands of that positional play e.g. skills
- know the energy systems used e.g. anaerobic and/or aerobic rest intervals etc.
- know the mechanism of injury so that in the final stages of

specific sport rehabilitation the injury must be stressed so as to replicate the original mechanism of injury.

Specific sports analysis

With information about the specific sport, the physiotherapist can then assess:

- the pathology and healing process of the injured part
- the requirements of the cardio-vascular system for that sport
- the specific sport fitness for that sport
- the specific rehabilitation for the injured part.

4 Organization of a Hydrotherapy Treatment Programme

If the athlete *cannot* perform normal movement in a weight bearing situation, then the swimming pool is an excellent environment to treat and train. The programme is organized in a similar way to the format of a training programme

- warm-up
- general mobilization exercises
- specific exercises related to the injured part
- interval work that replicates the demands of the sport cool down.

All athletes consider an injury to be a hindrance. Hydrotherapy offers many options in the specific rehabilitation and enhances the physiological and psychological well-being of the athlete.

Warm-up

- Warm-up is important in preparing the body both physiologically and psychologically for participating in the sporting activities. These principles of warm-up are well established for 'land' activities but are often forgotten in water activities. To assist the physiotherapist in determining these principles of warm-up in water, a list of guidlines are listed below:

Guidelines for warm-up in water

- In a warm-up, an athlete works heart rate (HR) between 40–60% depending upon the level of fitness. To calculate the athlete's maximal HR subtract the athlete's age from 220 then compute 40–60% of the maximal HR, e.g. 220 − 20 years' old = 200, 60% of 200 = 120 beats/minute. It is important to realize that the cardio-vascular system is subjected to stress while exercising in warm water of 34°C. At this temperature, the hydrostatic pressure on the stomach and chest forces the heart to work harder and care must be taken (Gleim, 1989). Because of this improved venous return, the stroke volume is increased thus resulting in a decreased cardiac output. Therefore, the above calculation should also include a subtraction of 8–10 beats to cater for this hydrostatic pressure. Every athlete must measure the HR before commencing the pool session and remeasure it during different phases of the session.

Activities for warm-up

● Swimming/walking/running in water can be excellent activities to prepare the body for more specific exercises especially related to the injured part. These activities are performed for a minimum of five minutes and up to ten minutes.

Depth of water increases the degree of difficulty of the activity (e.g. for running, the deeper the water, the more difficult the task).

● Walking and running activities vary in the degree of difficulty according to depth. In a recent study, Harrison and Bulstrode (1987) discuss the values of percentage weight bearing figures for different parts of the body. For instance, immersion to the level of supine C7 is approximately 8% weight bearing; immersion to the level of the xiphisternum is approximately 25–35% weight bearing and immersion to the level of anterior superior iliac is approximately 47–54% weight bearing. With these percentages of partial immersion, the physiotherapist can now accurately progress exercises according to these percentage weight bearing values.

General mobility exercises

● The athlete needs to maintain muscle strength and flexibility in the rest of the body that is uninjured. For instance, lower limb injuries require trunk and upper limb maintenance programmes. Swimming is an excellent conditioning exercise for maintenance and for exercising the muscles and joints of the entire body at one time. The number of laps recommended will depend upon the level of fitness of the athlete but

approximately between 10–20 minutes for aerobic maintenance is needed.

Specific exercises

- Hydrotherapy is of great value in the treatment of the various
injuries listed under the heading 'Common Conditions
Treated by Hydrotherapy' and all techniques may be needed
for specific work with the athlete.

Sports specific fitness: interval work

- Training in any sport should be specific to the energy demands
of the activity. Therefore hydrotherapy can be used to reproduce these sports specific energy requirements while the athlete
is injured. Usually most sports require an aerobic and/or
anaerobic component. The physiotherapist needs to assess
what the specific requirements are in the sport and then devise
a sports specific programme.

 For example, long distance runners require 90% aerobic and
10% anaerobic training. In direct contrast, sprint athletes
require 10% aerobic and 90% anaerobic training. Contact
team sports have different energy requirements depending
upon the specific positional play. For example, a defence
position usually requires a series of short sharp bursts of effort
60% aerobic and 40% anaerobic, whereas a centre position
usually requires 40% aerobic and 60% anaerobic work.

Cool down

- Cool down is the final stage of the rehabilitation training
programme and has both physiological and psychological
benefits. The athlete's heart rate needs to return to normal and
this can be achieved by 'winding down' and by repeating
some of the warm-up activities. These activities facilitate the
removal of lactic acid and may prevent muscle soreness.
Psychologically, the athlete has performed and achieved a
training programme which will enhance his confidence and
motivation.

This rehabilitation training programme has enabled the athlete to
achieve a specific hydrotherapy programme for the injured part and
maintained specific fitness for his sport.

5 Running in Water

In North America, running in water has become a popular method of treating and rehabilitating the injured athlete. Prokop (1985) cites several success stories of athletic coaches using the pools to rehabilitate their elite athletes. The most impressive case history was related to the middle distance runner Mary Decker. She developed a very sore Achilles tendon at the 1984 Olympic trials. She had approximately two weeks to recover for the Olympics. During this period, her coach allowed her to train only in the pool.

'She not only swam laps, but did running simulation exercises while suspended from the Aqua-Ark, a device with a polyurethane frame, one end of which rests on the side of the pool while the other end is supported in the water by plastic floats. Decker wore a life jacket that was tied to each leg of the Aqua-Ark, and moved her legs and arms as if she were actually running.' If the session was supposed to be a series of 440 seconds on land, then she would reproduce the same energy system training using the Aqua-Ark for about 60 seconds and then take about a two minute recovery ... 'With weights in her hands, the shoes on her feet and the altitude simulator attached, she had an excellent work out.' ... "How well this training worked for Decker is illustrated by the fact that only 10 days after she resumed track training, she set a world record for 2000 m.' (Prokop, 1985).

Gibson (1981) found that shallow water exercises are excellent for the rehabilitation and for training of athletes in inclement weather conditions. For the injured and uninjured athlete, running on the spot and running across the pool in three to four feet of water can yield maximum results, especially if the athlete breaks the surface of the water with the knee on each step.

Most of the literature discussing running in water relies on personal experience and successful case studies. However, one unpublished study by Hamer *et al.* (1984) investigated the comparison of non-weight bearing water running and treadmill running using cinematography as the objective measurement tool. They found that there are differences between non-weight bearing water running and treadmill running. The non-weight bearing water running action displays kinematic variations in the pattern of movement; the temporal aspects and the magnitude of the angular accelerations and velocities. This is obvious when assessing the stride rate of the non-weight bearing water running action which is shorter than treadmill running. Hamer *et al.* (1984) conclude that there is a difference between land and water running styles which implicates the difference in neuromuscular and physiological specificity of these two styles. However, non-weight bearing water running is recommended as part of a training programme and is especially beneficial for the injured athlete.

Recently, two studies have investigated the physiological responses to treadmill and water running. Bishop *et al.* (1989) tested seven non-injured athletes and compared their physiological responses to running on a treadmill and to running in water wearing a vest. Ventilation, oxygen uptake and respiratory quotient were significantly higher during treadmill running, whereas heart rate and perceived exertion were not significantly different for the two forms of exercise. Water running elicited a 36% lower metabolic cost than treadmill running despite the athlete's efforts to maintain a similar level of exertion. In contrast, Gleim and Nicholas (1989) found treadmill walking in water can double the oxygen cost of movement depending on the depth and speed, and the response to increasing speed is nonlinear. Water temperature affects the relationship of heart rate to maximal oxygen uptake at waist depth, suggesting that water temperature can add a significant thermal lead to the cardio-vascular system. Therefore, the metabolic and cardio-vascular demands of treadmill walking/jogging in water must be considered when used in rehabilitation programmes since greater external work results at much lower speeds than on land.

Hamer (1985) conducted another study which investigated water-running and the training effects on aerobic, anaerobic and muscular parameters following an eight week training interval training programme. This study involved nine male volunteer subjects who performed an eight week training/running sessions in shallow water of one metre. Overall, this study concluded that water running satisfies the principles of specificity of training for running activities and demonstrated improvement in both anaerobic and aerobic fitness. The implications of this study are very important for the physiotherapists in devising an exercise prescription programme.

Implications of the study:

1.   Interval water-running training is effective for the individual who needs to improve aerobic and anaerobic fitness.
2.   The acute and chronic responses, if water-running, are similar to those elicited during land-based running, so that the water environment can be used with confidence in either

short-term or long-term substitution of land-based running. This would allow the maintenance of cardiorespiratory and muscular fitness levels during injury to the locomotor system.

3. The improved cardio-vascular efficiency evident during standardized submaximal workloads while running in the water may have beneficial effects for 'at risk' populations. (Hamer, 1985).

Water running has been used as an experimental modality for the injured athlete. Only recently has water running captured the imagination of the researchers and with further objective investigations, the physiotherapist will be able to optimize the potential of water running in the rehabilitation of sports injuries.

REFERENCES

Bishop P. A., Frazier S., Smith J. *et al.* (1989). Physiological responses to treadmill and water running. *The Physician and Sportsmedicine.* **17**(2), 87–94.

Counsilman J. E. (1968). *The Science of Swimming.* Englewood Cliffs: Prentice-Hall.

Counsilman J. E. (1986). The role of the coach in training for swimming. *Clinics in Sports Medicine.* **5**(1), 3–7.

Evans P. (1980). The healing process at cellular level—a review. *Physiotherapy,* **66**(8), 256–259.

Fitch K. D. (1979). *Stress Fractures of the Lower Limb.* Perth: MTAA.

Fowler P. (1985). Rotation strength about the shoulder—establishment of internal to external strength ratios. *The New Zealand Journal of Sports Medicine.* **13**(3), 88–89.

Fricker P., Purdam C., Sweetenham B. *et al.* (1984). Swimmer's shoulder. *Sports Science and Medicine Quarterly.* **1**(2), 8–12.

Gibson K. (1981). Shallow water conditioning/rehabilitation for track *Scholastic Coach.* **50**(9), 52–58.

Gleim G. W., Nicholas J. A. (1989). Metabolic costs and heart rate responses to treadmill walking in water at different depths and temperatures. *American Journal of Sports Medicine.* **17**(2), 248–252.

Griepp J. F. (1985). Swimmer's shoulder: the influence of flexibility and weight training. *The Physician and Sportsmedicine.* **13**(8), 92–105.

Hamer P., Whittingham D., Spittles M. *et al.* (1984). *Cinematographical Comparison of Water Running to Treadmill Running.* (Unpublished paper.)

Hamer P. (1985). *Water—Running: Training Effects on Aerobic, Anaerobic Muscle Parameters following an Eight Week Interval Exercise*

Programme. Unpublished Honours Degree Thesis at the University of Western Australia.

Harrison R., Bulstrode S. (1987). Percentage weight bearing during partial immersion in the hydrotherapy pool. *Physiotherapy Practice.* 3(2), 60–63.

Hawkins R., Abrahams J. (1987). Impingement syndrome in the absence of rotator cuff tear. *Orthopedic Clinics of North America.* 18(3), 373–382.

Hawkins, R., Hobeikea P. (1983). Impingement syndrome in the athletic shoulder. *Clinics in Sports Medicine.* 2(2), 391–407.

Kennedy J. C., Hawkins R.J. (1974). Swimmer's shoulder. *The Physician and Sportsmedicine.* 2, 34–38.

Matheson J. A., Gerrard D. F. (1986). Some common overuse syndromes in swimmers. *The New Zealand Journal of Sports Medicine.* 14(1), 2–5.

McMaster, W. C. (1986). Painful shoulder in swimmers: a diagnostic challenge. *The Physician and Sportsmedicine.* 14(12), 108–122.

Noyes F. R., Paulos L., Mooar L.A. (1980). Knee sprains and acute knee hemarthrosis. *Physical Therapy.* 60(12), 1596–1601.

Penny J. N., Smith C. (1986). The prevention and treatment of swimmer's shoulder. *Canadian Journal of Applied Sports Science.* 5(3), 195–202.

Petersen L., Renstrom P. (1986). *Sports Injuries.* Australia: Methuen.

Prokop D. (1985). Water works. *Runner's World.* May, 59–71.

Rathbun J. B., McNab I. (1970). The microvascular pattern of the rotator cuff. *Journal of Bone and Joint Surgery.* 52B(3), 544–533.

Reid Campion M. (1985). *Hydrotherapy in Paediatrics.* Oxford: Heinemann Medical.

Richardson A. B., Jobe F. W., Collins H. R. (1980). The shoulder in competitive swimming. *American Journal of Sports Medicine.* 8(3), 159–163.

Rovere G. D., Nichols A. W. (1985). Frequency, Associated Factors, and Treatment of Breaststroker's Knee in Competitive Swimmers. *American Journal of Sports Medicine.* 13(2), 99–104.

Roy S., Irvin R. (1980). *Sports Medicine, Prevention, Evaluation, Management and Rehabilitation.* Englewood Cliffs: Prentice-Hall.

Sarrafian S. K. (1983). Gross and functional anatomy of the shoulder. *Clinical Orthopaedics and Related Research.* 173, 11–19.

Skinner A. T., Thomson A. M. (1983). *Duffield's Exercise in Water,* 3rd edn. London: Baillière Tindall.

Spencer J. D., Hayes K. C., Alexander I. J. (1984). Knee joint effusion and quadriceps reflex inhibition in man. *Arch Phy Med Rehabil.* 65(April), 171–177.

Stulberg S. D., Shulman K., Stuart S. *et al.* (1980). Breaststroker's knee: pathology, etiology and treatment. *American Journal of Sports Medicine.* 8(3), 164–171.

Vizsolyi P., Taunton J., Robertson G. (1987). Breaststroker's knee. An analysis of epidemiology and biomechanical factors. *American Journal of Sports Medicine.* **15**(1), 63–71.

FURTHER READING

Bolton E., Goodwin D. (1973). *Pool Exercises.* 4th edn. London: Churchill Livingstone.

Curwin S., Standish W. D. (1984). *Tendinitis: Its Etiology and Treatment.* Toronto: D. C. Heath and Co.

Davies B. A., Harrison R. A. (1988). *Hydrotherapy in Practice.* Edinburgh: Churchill Livingstone.

Fowler, P. J., Regan W. D. (1986). Swimming injuries of the knee, foot and ankle, elbow, and back. *Clinics in Sports Medicine.* **5**(1), 139–149.

Hay J. G. (1985). *The Biomechanics of Sports Techniques.* 3rd edn. London: Prentice-Hall International.

Kennedy J. C., Hawkins R. J., Krissoff, W. B. (1978). Orthopaedic manifestations of swimming. *American Journal of Sports Medicine.* **6**(6), 309–322.

Kennedy J. C. (1980). Breaststroker's knee: pathology, etiology and treatment. *American Journal of Sports Medicine.* **8**(3), 170–171.

McConnell J. (1986). The management of chondromalacia patellae: A long-term solution. *Australian Journal of Physiotherapy.* **32**(4), 215–223.

Reid D.C. (1986). Muscle imbalance around the swimmer's shoulder: summary. *The New Zealand Journal of Sports Medicine.* **14**(3), 23–24.

Richardson A. R. (1986). The biomechanics of swimming: the shoulder and knee. *Clinics in Sports Medicine.* **5**(1), 103–113.

Sarnaik A. P., Vohra M. P., Stirman S. W. (1986). Medical problems of the swimmer. *Clinics in Sports Medicine.* **5**(1), 47–63.

SECTION III

HEALTH PROMOTION

This section of the book is concerned with promoting health for individuals and in the community. It is the role of the physiotherapist to help in the restoration and maintenance of health and increasingly the psychosocial model is emerging. As Collins (1987) argues the physiotherapist may prove more effective in this role if he acts more as a partner than a prescriber in health care. This means that the physiotherapist must appreciate the definition of health and have an understanding of both the psychological and sociological dimensions of health. Collins (1987) quotes several definitions of health such as that of the World Health Organization (1978); that of Herzlich (1973) and a more simplistic definition—'the absence of disease'.

All definitions see the physical, mental and social well-being as important and interrelated and that these must be acceptable to the individual. Values, beliefs, attitudes and the environment will influence the individual and the community and it is vital in a psychosocial approach that the physiotherapist understands and is able to modify treatment and education programmes to allow for the psychological and social influences on the individual.

BENEFITS OF EXERCISE IN WATER

The benefits of exercise in general terms are widely known, but some physiotherapists may be less familiar with the benefits of exercise in water.

It is fun, refreshing, exhilarating and relaxing to participate in water activity. All degrees of exercise can be undertaken without weight bearing. There is no need to assume the upright position unless required. Muscular strength, physical fitness, and range of movement may be maintained and increased. Balance and coordination can be improved; pain decreased, swimming and safety skills acquired.

The psychological and social benefits are numerous, especially when activity takes place in a group.

The following chapters relate strongly to the psychosocial approach with an emphasis on maintaining and improving health and physical and mental well-being.

Collins M (1987). *Women's Health through Lifestages*, Sydney: Australian Physiotherapy Association.
Herzlich C., Graham D. (1974). *Health and Illness*, New York: Academic Press.

Hydrotherapy in the Childbearing Year

When a woman becomes pregnant she desires the best for her baby. If this means providing a healthy body in which the baby can develop it is likely that she will make some beneficial changes to her lifestyle. These changes may include a healthier diet, ensuring greater amounts of rest, relaxation and sleep and taking regular exercise.

If the pregnant woman is keen to start an exercise programme she should participate in a safe activity and one which she enjoys. Most pregnant women can continue with their normal activities including sport and other forms of exercise. For example, if the woman has been playing tennis in her pre-pregnant state she should be able to continue until her enlarging abdomen and other factors impose their limitations on her. She may enjoy cycling, walking or exercising in a group situation. Whatever the woman chooses, she should always check with her doctor first that there are no contra-indications to an exercise programme.

Exercise classes for pregnant women are traditionally held on land and provide the participants with all the benefits of a group situation. However, as the weeks progress the pregnant woman may find that her changing body is limiting her performance in some of the following ways. Swollen feet and ankles can make her feel clumsy, the pelvic floor is affected by repetitive bouncing movements, the pelvic joints may ache with the increasing weight, shortness of breath due to the enlarging uterus causing pressure against the diaphragm or she may feel generally uncomfortable and hot.

Exercise classes in water provide an excellent alternative and on entering the water the pregnant woman feels transformed. She can enjoy the support offered by the water and reap the other benefits from exercising in water which are discussed later in this chapter.

Aims of a water fitness class

1 To enhance the physiological and psychological well-being of women during pregnancy and childbirth.
2 To use water as an effective medium to counter the increasing weight of the pregnant woman.

Objectives of a water fitness class

1 Teach the basic physiology of pregnancy, the physical changes that occur in pregnancy and how the participants can reduce the risks of joint and soft tissue problems by performing exercises in a correct manner.
2 Inform the participants about the structure and function of the pelvic floor and how pregnancy and childbirth are potentially damaging to it.
3 Show that with improved cardio-vascular fitness and respiratory efficiency women should have increased confidence and endurance for labour.
4 Inform the participants about exercises which will help to decrease oedema and relieve varicose veins.
5 Teach the participants how to recognize and cope with tension by using appropriate relaxation techniques.

The pregnant woman will have her own reasons for exercising in water and some of these could be:

- to maintain or increase her fitness level
- to control her weight
- to help decrease backache
- to keep the abdominal muscles strong
- to decrease her swollen ankles and relieve her varicose veins
- to improve her posture
- to relieve any tension accumulated during the day
- to feel more comfortable.

By achieving one or more of these benefits the woman begins to feel and look better and experiences enhanced self esteem. Pregnancy often makes a women feel big, clumsy and unattractive so any positive factors which improve her body image are most important.

Water fitness can be performed individually or in a group situation. Many women prefer to exercise in a group because they feel more at ease and less self conscious; they receive peer group support and in turn become a resource and support person for others; they can socialize during a class, make new friends, compare aspects of their pregnancy with others and exercise with other pregnant women is more enjoyable.

Main Physical Benefits of Exercising in Water

Physical benefits of exercising in water accrue especially when the following points are considered.

1 There is a decreased amount of jarring on the joints of the body. As the amount of body submersion increases the percentage weight bearing decreases. For example, when submerged to the level of the xiphisternum the body experiences about 28% of actual body weight (Harrison and Bulstrode, 1987). Therefore, there is less strain on the weight bearing joints such as the lumbo-sacral area of the spine, pelvis and knees when exercising in water compared to exercising on land.

2 By exercising at an appropriate rate, the pregnant women can increase her cardio-vascular fitness and her respiratory efficiency which, in turn, make her feel fitter, stronger and more confident about coping with labour and delivery. It is possible to assess the woman's fitness by getting her to perform the '12 minute walk test'. To do this the pulse is taken and recorded, and then for 12 minutes she walks as many lengths or widths of the pool as she can. The distance covered is recorded, as is her pulse, on completion of the exercise. She keeps moving gently for five minutes and then her pulse is taken again when it should have returned to the starting rate.

3 60–70% of the maximum heart rate is normally a safe level of exertion for a pregnant woman. To calculate the maximum heart rate (MHR) the woman's age is subtracted from 220. Then to calculate the training or target heart rate, (THR) 65% of MHR is found. For example, if the woman is 26, her MHR is $220 - 26 = 194$. Her safe THR would be 65% of 194 which is 126 (Fox and Mathews, 1981). At the completion of the test, her pulse should not be above her estimated THR. If it is higher she should be advised to decrease her pace slightly. The woman's heart rate should be

below 100 within five minutes after stopping the exercise if the intensity is appropriate (Jopke, 1983).

4   The circulation is improved by increasing the venous return. When exercising in water the hydrostatic pressure on the legs acts as an additional pumping mechanism for the blood and lymphatic systems.

5   Hydrostatic pressure increases with the depth of the water (Pascal's Law). For example, if a woman is walking in 1.2 metres of water the hydrostatic pressure on her legs would be much greater than in 0.5 metres of water or floating on the surface. Therefore, swollen feet and ankles and varicose veins will be relieved during exercises in water.

6   When exercising on land the pregnant woman, especially during the summer, may find that high levels of activity can cause the maternal temperature to exceed 38°C. This rise in temperature may affect the developing fetus in the first trimester (Smith and Upfold, 1987).

   However, when exercising in cool water (26–30°C) body heat is evenly and effectively dissipated (Rocan, 1984) so maternal temperature is unlikely to exceed 37°C.

7   A greater amount of energy is expended while exercising in water. Froude (1984) and Zahm (1904) two scientists whose work was directed towards skin friction of a body in air and water, found that under similar conditions skin friction was proportional to the densities of the two mediums and that the skin friction in water was 790 times greater than air. This indicates therefore that a greater degree of energy is required to move in water (Reid Campion, 1985). This means that the muscles are working much harder to produce movement. As muscle strength and tone increase, the woman may notice her arms and legs are becoming firmer and more shapely.

8   Women need to be informed of the dangers of over working the abdominal muscles. In pregnancy these muscles are stretched over the ever enlarging uterus and if they are contracted too strongly the linea alba, the connective tissue between the two rectus abdominus muscles, may widen and cause a 'diastasis' of the recti (Noble, 1978).

9   Swimming and/or performing specific exercises provides an ideal way of exercising the abdominal muscles without 'over working' them. As abdominal tone is increased or maintained the woman's posture improves which, in turn,

makes her back less liable to postural strains (Mantle *et al.*, 1977).

10   In pregnancy the altered hormonal levels have a softening effect on the ligaments. This means that they stretch more easily making the joints more unstable and increasing the risk of injury (Noble, 1978). When exercising in water the movements are slower, more controlled and the joints are well supported. It is these factors which help decrease the risk of joint injury (Rocan, 1984).

Points To Consider in Water Fitness Programmes

There are two major points that have to be considered in water fitness programmes—backpain and fatigue.

Back pain is a common complaint during pregnancy. Three main areas are at risk; the sacro-iliac and pubic symphysis joints, the lumbo-sacral region and the thoracic area. The sacro-iliac joints and the pubic symphysis are usually very stable joints but during pregnancy the hormone, relaxin, softens the ligaments of these joints and any disruptions to either of these joints has a destabilizing effect on the bony pelvic ring. Low back pain is often caused by the postural changes brought about by the enlarging uterus. The lumbar lordosis increases and there is often a compensatory thoracic kyphosis which puts extra strain on the muscles and ligaments of the vertebral column (Mantle *et al.*, 1977).

The physiotherapist must educate women regarding pain and strain that can arise from poor posture, prolonged postures and faulty lifting techniques. The pregnant woman should be shown how to perform pelvic rocking to relieve discomfort, to change her posture frequently and adopt safe lifting procedures.

The physiotherapist may need to advise the pregnant woman on any exercises that increase her back pain. For example, limiting the range of leg movements if pain is caused in either the sacro-iliac or pubic symphysis joints. [The woman may also benefit from the wearing of an abdominal or lumbar support such as the 'Owata Obi' or a 'Fembrace'].

In the all encompassing and supportive medium of water and in water that is warm, back pain is often relieved. It is possible to carry out back pain relieving measures and modifying swimming strokes which allows the pregnant woman to continue an activity without increasing back pain. Fatigue must be taken into account when exercising in water. Therefore, a water fitness class should be treated in the same way as any other exercise class in respect to the careful monitoring of the progression of exercise.

As so much more energy is expended when exercising in water the physiotherapist must advise new participants on the dangers of over working. It is easy not to notice fatigue, overdo the exercises and suffer from the effects for days afterwards. Before starting any exercise, participants should be advised regarding the signs of fatigue which are tiredness during or after an exercise period, the need to take a rest after the class or increased Braxton Hicks contractions.

Braxton Hicks contractions are the painless contractions of the uterus during pregnancy (Williams, 1985). As the pregnancy nears full-term (40 weeks) these contractions tend to increase in frequency. However, if a pregnant woman is overworking this can also increase these contractions and the woman should take heed and decrease her activity level.

Screening and Safety of Participants

The screening and the safety of the participants is of paramount importance. Ideally the participants should complete a consent form before joining any class. If there are any contra-indications to the pregnant woman exercising, the physiotherapist must know about these, thus it is essential that the woman's doctor completes a consent form supplying details of her blood pressure and any other relevant obstetric history.

The participants must be advised to stop exercising if they experience any pain. They should slow down or stop if they feel tired or unwell in any way. They should avoid exercising if they are recovering from an illness such as influenza. They should not enter the water if they have a skin, ear, nose or throat or urinary tract infection. If they feel any dizziness or nausea they should also stop exercising and leave the pool informing the physiotherapist that they are doing so. They should be discouraged from holding their breath while performing any exercise as this can cause an unnecessary rise in intra-thoracic pressure which may lead to a decreased blood flow back to the heart or the placenta.

Water temperature

The temperature of the water is important. Below 25°C participants may complain of the cold and temperatures over 34°C tend to make pregnant women feel nauseous and very tired. The ideal water temperature would be between 26–30°C, though temperatures between 30–32°C are advocated by Vleminckx (1988) and it is easier to promote relaxation in warmer water. In lower temperature ranges, exercise would need to be carried out more rapidly to prevent heat loss to the water.

Depth of water

The ideal depth of the water would be to the level of the xiphisternum. As the depth in most commercial pools is usually 0.9–1.2 metres at the shallow end, the physiotherapist should endeavour to exercise the participants in an area of the pool where the water is deep enough to cover the abdomen. In this way the pregnant uterus is at all times fully supported by the water and any bouncing effects minimized. However, if the depth of water increases to above the level of the xiphisternum vertical balance is threatened.

Format of a Water Fitness Class

The format of a water fitness class is similar to other exercise classes in that the different components of the programme are included. For example, the participants *warm-up* before they *stretch*. Once the major muscle groups have been stretched the *aerobic* component follows to increase the efficiency of the cardio-vascular and respiratory systems. *Strengthening* exercises are important for the main muscle groups and to complete the programme the participants should have a *cool down stretch* followed by some *relaxation*.

Suggested exercises for a water fitness class

The pulse is taken at the start of the class and again after the aerobic component. A final pulse is taken five minutes after the second reading to gauge the participants recovery rate.

WARM-UP

- Walking forwards—two lengths
- Walking sideways—two lengths

- Walking sideways with a 'cross-over'—two lengths (Zorba the Greek step)
- Walking backwards—two lengths
- Jogging forwards—two lengths
- Jogging backwards—two lengths (Jogging is only done if the water is at ideal depth i.e. xiphisternum level).

If the physiotherapist has chosen to work across the width of the pool to maintain the optimum depth of water for the group, the above mentioned lengths would become widths.

Strong swimmers may wish to swim their *warm-up* instead of walking and can use a variety of strokes for this component providing their stroke technique does not cause any ligamentous strain. For example, the width of the breaststroke kick should be decreased if the woman complains of any pain in the pubic symphysis joint and also when she is swimming breaststroke she should be encouraged to keep her head down as low as possible to minimize hyperextension of the lower back.

STRETCHING

Before starting the programme the participants should be advised not to 'over do' their stretches because it is possible to damage the ligaments and strain the joints.

Shoulder stretches

- With the hands clasped in front of the body and the feet 0.5 metres apart, slowly lift the arms upwards over the head. Hold this for eight seconds then release. Remind the participants not to 'arch' the back beyond its natural curve. Repeat this stretch three times.

- With the hands clasped behind the body and the feet 0.5 metres apart, slowly lift the arms upwards. Hold this for eight seconds. Repeat this stretch three times.

- Standing with the feet 0.5 metres apart. Right hand towards the back of neck, left hand between the shoulder blades. Try to grasp the fingers of the left hand with the fingers of the right hand.

Hold this for eight seconds then release. Repeat this stretch three times on each side.

Quadriceps stretch (Fig. 9.1a)

With a partner, grasp the partner's right forearm, hold your own left ankle and slowly stretch left heel to left buttock. Hold this for eight seconds and then gently release this three times each side changing the arm hold with the partner as appropriate.

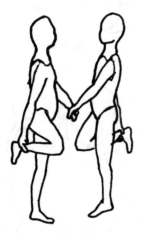

Fig. 9.1a

Hamstring stretch (Fig. 9.1b)

With a partner, grasp the partner's right forearm, holding the left knee and gently pull it up and slightly outwards. Hold this for eight seconds and then slowly release. Repeat this three times on each side.

Calf stretch (Fig. 9.1c)

With arms straight and hands against the partner's hands at shoulder level and feet in walking position, gently lean towards the partner feeling the stretch in the calf muscles. It is important to maintain the pelvic tilt during this exercise so as not to increase the lumbar lordosis which can cause ligament strain.

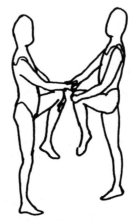

Fig. 9.1b

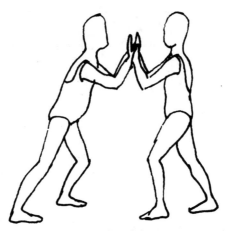

Fig. 9.1c

Side lunge (Fig. 9.1c)

With arms straight and hands against the partner's hands at shoulder level, feet about shoulder width apart, lean towards the right. The right knee flexes and the left inner thigh stretches. Hold this for eight seconds and then slowly release. Repeat three times on each side. The partner mirrors the action by moving to her left.

Rotation stretch (Fig. 9.1e)

Back to back with the partner, about 0.5 metre away and feet 0.5

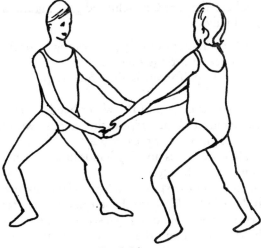

Fig. 9.1d

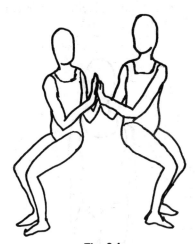

Fig. 9.1e

metre apart. Bend knees when turning to touch each other's hands. Hold the stretch for eight seconds. Repeat this stretch three times on each side.

AEROBICS

This section lasts for 12–15 minutes starting off gently, building up at a pace where the THR is achieved and maintained and then lowered gradually.

- Alternate heel raises, gradually progressing to jogging on the spot lifting the knees a little higher.
- Jogging four steps forwards then four steps back. Repeat this eight times.
- With both hands on top of the water bend the right knee up to touch the hands and then repeat the exercise with the left knee. Repeat this eight times on each side.
- As the right knee bends up, clap hands underneath it. Repeat this eight times on each side.
- While jogging on the spot, touch the right ankle with the right hand and the left ankle with the left hand. Then touch the right ankle with the left hand and *vice versa*. Touch the right heel with the right hand and the left heel with the left hand. Touch the right heel with the left hand and *vice versa*. Touch the right ankle with the left hand and then the left heel with the right hand and *vice versa*. Repeat all the movements eight times on each side (see Fig. 9.2).

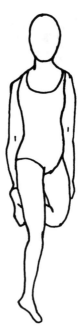

Fig. 9.2

The physiotherapist can use a variety of equipment in the aerobic exercises for example, rubber volley balls, balloons and hoops.

- Participants form a circle and whilst gently jogging on the spot use both hands to throw the balls around the circle in a clockwise direction. This exercise can be altered by:

(a) changing direction frequently
(b) using only the right hand
(c) using only the left hand
(d) passing the ball around body before throwing it on
(e) passing the ball under one leg before throwing it on
(f) pushing the ball under the water five times before throwing it on.

- Participants form a circle, facing in a clockwise direction, the ball is tossed carefully over the head for the person behind to catch. This exercise can be altered by:

(a) turning to the right before throwing the ball on
(b) turning to the left before throwing the ball on.

It is important to remind participants to bend their knees as they turn so as not to strain their backs; also to keep jogging while waiting for the next ball to come.

- The participants hold hands in a circle formation and side step to the right, e.g. step with the right foot approximately 0.5 metres to the right and then bring the left foot to touch the right foot. After approximately 30 seconds change direction. It will be appreciated by the participants how hard it is to work against the flow of water initially. Alter this exercise by:

(a) side stepping with a cross-over (Zorba the Greek dance step.)
(b) walking backwards and then changing direction
(c) jogging four steps into the middle and four steps back out again.

Easy dance routines can be included into the aerobic component for example:

- With a partner two metres away jog towards each other and touch the right hand, jog backwards away from each other. Continue this routine by touching:

(a) left hands then both hands
(b) right elbows, left elbows and then both

(c) right shoulders, left shoulders then both (back to back)
(d) right foot, left foot then both feet
(e) right knee, left knee then both
(f) right hip, left hip then both (back to back)
(g) right arm swing, left arm swing then swing partner with both arms.
(h) 'Do-ce-Do' arms folded jog towards the partner and pass to the right and jog backwards to starting position.

STRENGTHENING EXERCISES

It is important when performing strengthening exercises to guard against fatigue. Repetitions should be kept to approximately eight and alternating between arm and leg exercises will also guard against this factor. If the participants are feeling at all cold encourage them to jog two lengths after each four sets of exercises.

When exercising the arms it is important that the shoulders are submerged for if the shoulders and arms are out of the water the participants may as well be exercising on land! To keep the shoulders submerged the participants should be in crouch walk standing.

● With the arms at the side of the body at shoulder level, the palms facing inwards and fingers together, sweep arms forwards so that the hands meet in front of the body. Pronate the forearms so that the palms face outwards and then sweep the arms backwards to the starting position. To progress the exercise the movement is performed more rapidly.

Leg exercises to develop muscle strength in the hip flexors, hip extensors, quadriceps and hamstrings

● Standing on the left leg push the right leg forwards keeping the knee straight then push it backwards in a pendulum type movement. It is important to maintain the pelvic tilt so as not to increase the lumbar lordosis, this exercise can be modified in the following way to prevent this.

Standing with the back against the side of the pool, lift the right leg up keeping the knee straight then return to starting position. Next stand approximately 0.5 metre from the pool side facing the wall holding on with both hands. Push the right leg backwards then return to the starting position.

- Standing on the left leg lift the right leg out to the side keeping the knee straight then return to the starting position. Repeat with the left leg.
- Arms circling backwards as in backstroke and then circling forwards as in freestyle (see Fig. 9.3a).
- Standing on left leg circle right leg backwards then circle it forwards. Repeat with left leg.
- Arms performing breaststroke whilst the participant is in crouch walk standing. This arm exercise can also be performed whilst the participant is walking with bent knees so that the shoulders remain submerged.
- Standing on the left leg, lift right leg forwards and then out to the side. Lean forwards as the leg swings to the back and then return the leg to the starting position. Reverse this movement by going backwards then to the side and then to the front and down. Repeat with the left leg (*see* Figs. 9.3b,c).

If balancing is a problem, stand side on to the pool side and hold the bar with the inside hand.

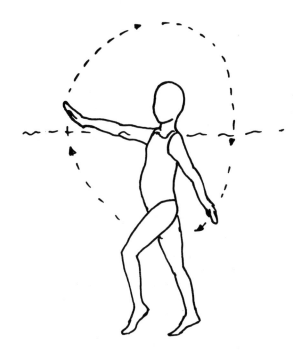

Fig. 9.3a

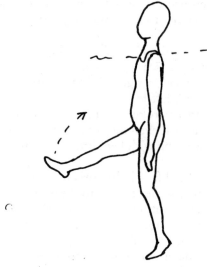

Fig. 9.3b

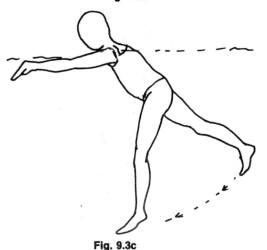

Fig. 9.3c

Push ups for the arms and shoulders

- Stand facing the side of the pool 0.5 metre away, hands holding the edge. Lean forwards and let the elbows bend and then push away. The heels may be kept flat if an extra stretch on the calf muscles is wanted. Participants should be reminded to decrease the lumbar lordosis by performing a pelvic tilt.

Leg kicks for the buttocks and legs

● Hold on to the sides of the pool with one hand higher than the other. This helps reduce the lumbar lordosis. Kick the legs alternately up and down keeping the knees straight and the heels just breaking the surface. This can also be performed holding on to a kick board (*see* Fig. 9.3d,e).

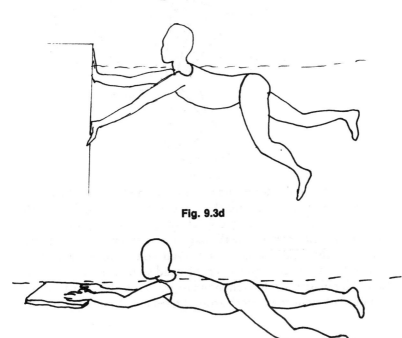

Fig. 9.3d

Fig. 9.3e

Cycling for the legs

● With the back to the side of the pool hold on to the bar (Fig. 9.3f) and move the legs in a cycling movement. This can also be performed by floating on back with a kickboard held to the chest. A kickboard can be used for strengthening the arms and shoulders.

    With one hand on each end of the board push it down by straightening the arms then slowly let it rise to the surface. Then push the board away from the body and then pull it back towards the body. (Make sure the board is fully submerged and vertical in the water to offer maximum resistance.)

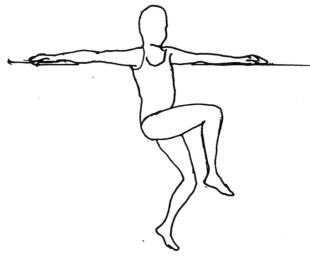

Fig. 9.3f

- Mobilize the shoulder joints by passing the kickboard over the head and downwards with the right hand, grasping it with the left hand which has come backwards and up towards the shoulder blades. Complete the exercise by extending the left arm bringing the board down and around and then in front of the body. Bend the left elbow over the head so board is between the shoulder blades for the right hand to grasp. i.e. the board is doing a figure of eight movement around the shoulders (see Fig. 9.3g).

Knee bends for strengthening the quadriceps

Keep the back straight and the heels flat while the knees bend and then straighten slowly.
- Pelvic floor exercises. With the legs slightly apart. Close the back and front passages—draw them up inside—hold this *SQUEEZE* and *LIFT* for five to ten seconds—let go *SLOWLY*.

Cool Down

- Standing with feet 0.5 metres apart and knees comfortably bent circle the hips in a clockwise direction. Change direction. (Belly dancing.)
- Pelvic rocking. Standing with feet 0.5 metre apart and knees bent comfortably tilt the pubic bones towards the chin. Then com-

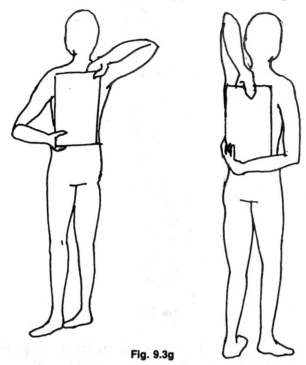

Fig. 9.3g

bine this exercise with a pelvic floor contraction i.e. *SQUEEZE* as the pubic bones tilt upwards (see Fig. 9.4). Pelvic rocking is an excellent exercise for relieving backache and can be performed in many positions.

- Standing with knees comfortably bent, feet apart and arms out in front of body. With both palms facing towards the right slowly sweep the arms to the right of the body. Move the hands so both palms are facing to the left and sweep the arms to the left of the body.

Breathing exercises

- Standing comfortably with the arms by the sides of body. Breathe in as the arms are lifted above the head, breathe out as the arms come down.
- Standing comfortably with arms by sides of body. Breathe in as the right arm is lifted over head as trunk flexes to the left. Breathe out as the body straightens and the arm comes down. Repeat to

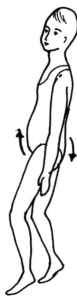

Fig. 9.4

the other side. These last two exercises should be performed slowly so that the participants do not 'overbreathe'.

Physiological relaxation (Mitchell, 1987) is the favoured technique for relaxation used by physiotherapists in Western Australia. It is mostly taught in preparation for childbirth classes, physiotherapy classes and other groups where learning to cope with stress is one of the main aims.

This method can be used to obtain relaxation of the whole body or just specific areas. It is based on the physiological laws of reciprocal muscle action, i.e., when one muscle group contracts the opposite group relaxes. The method is easy to teach, easy to learn and once learnt it can be used in many everyday stressful situations.

Physiological relaxation can provide the physiotherapist with an ideal way to end a water fitness class. If total body relaxation is wanted the participants need flotation devices to support their hips and shoulders. Once the women are comfortably supported the physiotherapist takes them through the different muscle groups in a special sequence until a 'position of ease' is achieved.

To use physiological relaxation the physiotherapist needs to know the exact orders that are given to each muscle group and these orders should not vary. These orders are given to each area in turn and they are:

1. To move the part into the reverse of the position of stress—i.e. 'the position of ease'.
2. To stop doing this movement.
3. To be aware of the new position.

Changes in body position and awareness are learnt quickly and by frequent practice greater depths of relaxation are obtained in a shorter period of time.

If there are not enough flotation devices available the physiotherapist can teach physiological relaxation in standing quite successfully. However, some participants may prefer to relax by leisurely swimming a few lengths before leaving the pool or having a discussion. A comfortable position for pregnant women is standing with knees and hips flexed, feet apart, forearms resting on a kickboard and slowly swirling from left to right.

INDIVIDUAL EXERCISE PROGRAMME

The above exercises can all be used on an individual basis except for those aerobic activities where a partner or group is needed. All the stretches with a partner can be adapted either by balancing carefully or using the side of the pool on which to hold for stability.

POSTNATAL EXERCISE CLASS

The postnatal period is considered to be 0–6 months postpartum. As soon as the lochia has ceased, the new mother could be encouraged to take part in a water fitness class. New mothers combine well with pregnant women and enhance the peer group support with their recent experiences and insight.

Water is a comfortable medium for the postpartum woman in which to exercise. She benefits from all the same factors mentioned earlier.

The physiotherapist should advise the postnatal woman that for several months after delivery her hormone level can continue to affect the ligaments, keeping them soft and prone to over stretching. This factor increases the risk of joint instability and possible damage. Therefore, the postnatal woman must be advised about

the dangers of overstretching and performing exercises too stren-
uously.

The new mother's pelvic floor may be considerably weakened
from the pregnancy and delivery and any 'bouncy' exercise movements on a hard surface could further weaken these structures. As
mentioned earlier exercising in water reduces the jarring effect on
the pelvic floor and weight bearing joints. Therefore the postnatal
woman would benefit from being able to exercise without doing
any damage to these important muscles.

The lactating woman's breasts are larger and heavier and this can
make exercising on land extremely uncomfortable. However, this is
not a problem when in the water provided the breasts are submerged.

Having new mothers in the class also gives the physiotherapist
an ongoing opportunity to enquire about her physical well-being
and arrange treatment for any physical problems if it is needed, for
example, back pain, diastasis of the abdominal recti, stress,
incontinence and dyspareunia.

MUSIC FOR EXERCISING

Using music in a water fitness class can enhance the feeling and
mood of the participants making the time pass quickly and
enjoyably. Music also adds rhythm to the exercises which is
important and often the women will sing along with the music
which can further enhance their enjoyment of the class. However, if
there is a lot of noise in the pool area from other users, the
physiotherapist may find that the music is creating a confusing
atmosphere and in that case using her own voice for instruction in a
rhythmical way may be more effective.

For the *warm-up* some lively music with a strong beat is
inspiring. *Stretching* is best done to slow and gentle music. The
aerobic segment needs happy, dance-type music, but care should be
taken that the beat is not too fast. (Exercises take longer to perform
in water than they do on land.) The *strengthening* component
requires slower music than the *aerobic* component and for the *cool
down* and *stretch* gentle music should be used.

It is advantageous to pre-record music onto one tape to suit the
class format as this enhances the smooth running and enjoyment of
the class.

SWIMMING IN PREGNANCY

Swimming may form part of the antenatal water fitness class but a pregnant woman may wish to pursue swimming over and above that as a means of maintaining fitness. If so, the choice of a suitably heated pool is important; excessive fatigue and exhaustion should be avoided and the precautions given earlier in this chapter need to be observed.

As a general rule swimmers are advised not to swim alone and this golden rule should apply to the pregnant woman. It's more enjoyable to exercise with a companion and swimming is no exception.

Swimming is considered to be the finest exercise, and because it is an aerobic exercise carried out in a non-weight bearing situation it is most appropriate for the pregnant woman (Pirie, 1987). Swimming involves large muscle groups combined with breathing control, rhythmical movements and if the swimming strokes are conducted at a slow or moderate pace, proves relaxing.

All four limbs are used to propel the body through the water, the major effort coming from the arms. A strong stable trunk provides the base from which the limbs may move in all the strokes; i.e. breaststroke, freestyle, backstroke, sidestroke and butterfly.

Each pregnant woman who can swim may continue to use her usual stroke or strokes, but she should be advised to report any pain or stresses on her joints. The most likely joints to suffer are the spine, sacro-iliac, hips and knees. Breaststroke may place undue strain on the spine due to the degree of extension required. Keeping the face lower in the water may reduce the extension of the spine but where back pain persists this modification may not give sufficient relief. A change of stroke is advisable.

The kick into extension/abduction with some external rotation may compress the sacro-iliac joints and place rotatory stress on the hip and knee joints. As an alternative the woman may swim freestyle or backstroke.

If back pain is not relieved a woman should be advised to swim using backstroke. If necessary, a bilateral arm movement that takes the upper limbs low over the water to shoulder height where the arms enter the water and pull to the sides of the body, may be useful (Reid Campion, 1985). This action reduces any rotation of the trunk and combined with a gentle backstroke kick is the least stressful of all the strokes. It can also be used, with some flotation equipment if necessary, for non-swimmers.

All strokes can be modified if they cause problems. Modifications may be small but will allow a woman to continue swimming in comfort. As the pregnancy advances the weight changes of the second and third trimesters may make swimming, especially in the prone position, difficult. Breathing is less easy on the stomach and thus a change of stroke that involves the supine position is advisable.

Swimming produces an aerobic effect even when carried out at a moderate pace. There are many advantages to swimming when pregnant and few disadvantages. Avoiding too hot or too cold water is recommended and the precautions given for the water exercise programme apply. Sibley *et al.* (1981) found that a swimming conditioning programme may well counteract any tendencies to diminished fitness during pregnancy. Their research also found that physiological processes such as maternal blood pressure and pulse remained within acceptable levels and the fetus was similarly unaffected by the swimming activity of its mother.

Artal (1986) suggests that the non-swimmer may even learn to swim during pregnancy. However, competitive swimming may only be acceptable in the first trimester (Diddle, 1984) a view that contrasts with that of Pirie (1987) who advises against it suggesting that the fetus may be deprived of an adequate oxygen supply.

SWIMMING POSTNATALLY

The postpartum woman may resume swimming following the 6 week medical examination. All modifications of strokes and other precautionary measures apply in the early months following the birth of her child, but the amount of activity can be steadily increased as the months pass. Since the hormone *relaxin* is still present in the body up to six months postpartum, care should be taken not to stress joints and ligaments, thus a gradual increase in the level of activity is advisable.

OTHER AQUATIC SPORTS

Diddle (1984) and Pirie (1987) are amongst the authors who consider that other aquatic sport such as diving, scuba diving and water skiing are potentially dangerous to the mother and the infant she carries and should be avoided antenatally and it would appear sensible to avoid these activities for a period of time postnatally whilst the body tissues are still at risk.

REFERENCES

Artal R., Wiswell R. A. eds. (1986). *Exercise in Pregnancy*, Baltimore: Williams & Wilkins.

Collins M. (1987). *Women's Health through lifestages*, Sydney: Australian Physiotherapy Association.

Diddle A. W. (1984). Interrelationship of pregnancy and athletic performance. *Journal of the Tennessee Medical Association*, 77(5), 256–69.

Fox E. L., Mathews D. K. (1981). *The Physiological Basis of Physical Education and Athletics*, New York: CBS College Publishing.

Harrison R., Bulstrode F. (1987). Percentage weight bearing during partial emersion in a hydrotherapy pool. *Physiotherapy Practices*, 3(2), 60–63.

Herzlich C., Graham D. (1974). *Health & Illness*, New York: Academic Press.

Jopke T. (1983). Pregnancy—A time to exercise judgement. *The Physician and Sports Medicine*, 2(7).

Mantle M. J., Greenwood R. M., Curry H. L. F. (1977). Backache in pregnancy. *Rheumatology Rehabilitation*, 16, 95–101.

Mitchell L. (1987). *Simple Relaxation: The Mitchell Method of Physiological Relaxation for Easing Tension*. London: John Murray.

Noble E. (1978). *Essential Exercises for the Childbearing Year*. London: John Murray.

Pirie L. (1987). *Pregnancy and Sports Fitness*. Tucson: Fisher Books.

Reid Campion M. (1985). *Hydrotherapy in Paediatrics*. Oxford: Heinemann Medical.

Rocan S. (1984). Aqua fitness — an overview, *Fitness Leader*, March, 2, 7.

Sibley L., Ruhling R. O. Cameron-Foster J. *et al.* (1981). Swimming and physical fitness during pregnancy. *Journal of Nurse-Midwifery*, 26(6), 3–12.

Smith M., Upfold J. (1987). Avoid heat stress in early pregnancy *Australian Doctor Weekly*, 10,7,87, 15.

Vleminckx I. M. (1988). Pregnancy and recovery: the aquatic approach. In *Obstetrics and Gynaecology* (McKenna J. ed.), Edinburgh: Churchill Livingstone.

Williams M., Booth D. (1985). *Antenatal Education*. New York: Churchill Livingstone.

WHO (1978). Primary health care In *Declaration of Alma Ata Primary Health Care*. Geneva: WHO.

Aqua Relaxation for Mothers and Babies

A mother with a newborn child needs to spend almost all of her time and energy caring for the child (Whiteford and Polden, 1984).

Extra energy and patience are immediately required with the onset of problems that may occur during infancy. It is in such situations that tension levels rise. Tension may be due to changes in the baby or in the mother (Cobb, 1980) and can interfere with the dynamics of the family and household. The most beneficial aspect of relaxation is in relieving these tensions. Gentle swimming in warm water can promote relaxation and early childhood is the optimal time to learn to relax and enjoy water (Madders, 1979).

AIMS

The overall aim of the programme is to reduce tension in both mother and child. It has been found that a group situation is beneficial but the group should not be too large. Approximately four to six mothers and their infants is suitable; to some extent the size of the group depends on the size and shape of the pool, but too large a number of participants is not advised.

Primary Aims

Specifically the aims of relaxation sessions are to:

● promote relaxation in the mother and child
● promote mother and child bonding
● increase the child's sleeping time
● provide a 'self' support situation

Secondary Aims

Certain secondary aims result from the child's activity with the mother in the water. These are:

- the promotion of head control
- the promotion of head and truncal righting reactions
- the promotion of sensory-motor development

Relaxation

The therapeutic qualities of warm water for exercise as well as for relaxation have been well documented.

Immersion of a person in warm water aids relaxation as does the support given by buoyancy (Skinner and Thomson, 1983) and the apparent weightlessness that is experienced (Harris and McInnes, 1963).

Leboyer (1975) subjectively reported the effectiveness of warm water immersion inducing a calming effect on the newborn.

Other authors, Wilson and Kasch (1963) and Kraus (1973) cited by Reid Campion (1985) have noted the sedative effect of warm water and research by Euler and Soderberg (1956) quoted by Harris (1978) report the reduction of muscle tone brought about by warm water.

Anxiety

In a study of the effect of hydrotherapy on anxiety Levine (1984) found, both subjectively and with electromyographic measures (EMG) a reduction in anxiety with only 15 minutes of hydrotherapy. Although no long-term assessment was made this study suggests that immersion in warm water can have a significant short-term effect on anxiety.

Articles and studies concerned with the influence of anxiety on the mother–infant bond vary in their discussions concerning anxiety and its effects on the mother–infant relationship (Barnett *et al.*, 1987; Mertin, 1986). Most agree that anxiety does affect the mother–infant relationship to some degree. In so far as 'the mother–infant relationship' is an ongoing developmental process rather than a postpartum event occurring in the first few days after birth

(Mertin, 1986) it seems important to reduce anxiety and to ensure every opportunity to maximize the mother–infant relationship.

The reduction in the mother's anxiety level usually means that she is more likely to cope with her child's sleep pattern.

Self support

Mothers in the group find comfort and help in knowing that someone else is experiencing similar problems.

Head control

The importance of developing head control is recognized in this programme. The Halliwick approach to head control (Reid Campion, 1985) is used. Activities which facilitate head control are chosen and the appropriate songs and rhymes are employed. The actions forming the programme are:

- jumping
- swaying i.e. deviating laterally whilst in the vertical position
- moving from the vertical position to supine and back to the vertical

Head and truncal righting reactions

Head and truncal righting reactions can be promoted using modified activities as suggested by Reid Campion (1985). Full explanations of these techniques and the appropriate holds are provided by that author, however some of these holds can be seen in Figs 10.1, 10.2, 10.3, 10.4.

Sensory-motor Development

A motor output requires a sensory input. Piaget's (1963) theory of development emphasizes the importance of the development of the sensory-motor system. The brain responds to messages it receives from the environment and the body's relationship to that environment as well as to internal factors such as body parts in relation to another body part and to the state of muscle tone. Such sensory feedback requires an intact sensory system and is provided by the proprioceptors in joints, muscles and tendons, in the skin, eyes and ears resulting in the production of appropriate reactions in the motor system (Shepherd, 1980).

In the pool various senses are stimulated to promote sensory-motor integration. The senses affected are:

- tactile
- vestibular
- auditory
- proprioception

Tactile sensation is stimulated by the water which is all encompassing but also by contact with the mother's body. Movement through water creates turbulence and promotes body awareness especially distally in the limbs. The turbulence created by others moving in the water further aids tactile awareness. The vestibular system is stimulated by the 'jumping' up and down, the swaying from side to side and going round in circles in some of the activities.

The songs that are sung in the activities provide stimulation to the auditory system at the same time as developing rhythm which further promotes relaxation for mother and child. The proprioceptive system receives information from muscles, joints and tendons and the resistance or impedance to movement provided by water stimulates proprioception.

CRITERIA FOR THE AQUA-RELAXATION PROGRAMME

Certain criteria for the programme have been formulated. It has been found valuable to utilize a group situation, but in some instances this needs to be varied to suit particular situations.

- It is of paramount importance that the mother and her child have had their six weeks postpartum examination by their doctor. There should be no contra-indications to hydrotherapy.
- Mothers suffering from postnatal depression should be seen on an individual basis until the mother and physiotherapist are happy with the progress at which time the mother normally joins the group.
- The number in the group is largely determined by the size and the shape of the pool, but whatever the dimensions of the pool small

groups are always advisable. There must be adequate space for the mothers to float; where large numbers are involved the situation may not be sufficiently relaxing.

- In regard to the infants the criteria is that they must wear snugly fitting pants.

Referrals

New or expectant mothers are made aware of the aqua-relaxation programme through the hospital and antenatal classes or those run by private physiotherapists, through antenatal and postnatal classes; by the maternity ward physiotherapist and notices displayed in doctor's surgeries. However, it appears that the majority hear of the programme from friends and relatives. Some women are referred by Infant Health nurses, others by private physiotherapists and doctors.

The most common reasons for referral are:

- poor sleeping
- colic
- mother not coping
- feeding problems
- other medical problems
- unsettled baby
- postnatal blues
- mother wishing child to get used to water

Assessment

A subjective history should be taken including the following items:

- details of the pregnancy
- details of the labour
- feeding and sleeping behaviour of the infant
- attendance at antenatal classes
- the type of relaxation taught
- the referral source
- the mother's swimming ability

In passing, the mother is asked about pelvic floor exercises, knowledge and practice. Objectively, a brief developmental assessment of the child should be carried out. Age appropriate milestones are assessed particularly the level of head control. In the pool the mother's reaction to the water is observed and recorded later, as well as her confidence in handling the baby and the baby's reaction to immersion.

Procedure

Prior to the first pool session it is advisable to offer the mother the opportunity of discussing baby massage, the advantages of the technique and if desired the chance to practise it.

Baby massage in different forms has been used in other cultures for centuries. However, in our society touching comes less easily. A physiotherapist who is trained in massage and with 'permission to touch' is the ideal person to teach mothers how to massage their baby. When used correctly it becomes part of the total handling of the baby and provides the tactile sensation to the skin that is so important in a child's development. Baby massage is a loving and caring way of helping babies and young children to feel that the world is a pleasurable, familiar safe place. It can prove relaxing for the mother as well. For the baby with special needs baby massage can have beneficial effects (Auckett, 1981).

Similar effects can be brought about by water; the child and its mother appreciate the all encompassing nature of water, the uniform pressure and the warmth all helping to provide tactile sensation and relaxation. The pool sessions involve 15 minutes of total relaxation for the mothers whilst the babies are cared for by others. The women are usually supported by neck, pelvic and ankle rings, but they use whatever flotation equipment they find comfortable. Music, which enhances relaxation is played and the mothers are encouraged to use the relaxation technique with which they are familiar. If they have no particular method, physiological relaxation is taught (Mitchell, 1987).

Following the relaxation period, in a water temperature of approximately 34°C (93.2°F) the babies are brought to the pool and join their mothers. Initially, the infants are introduced into the water very slowly the mother holding her child close to her and attempting to maintain eye contact. It is essential that the child feels secure and this security can be provided by the mother's arms and closeness and from the sensation of the fluid environment which is similar to that experienced prenatally (Reid Campion, 1985).

The time spent in the pool by the infant needs to be carefully monitored as their thermo-regulatory mechanisms are not as well developed as those of adults (Quinn, 1981). For the first visit, the time the child usually spends in the bath at home is used as the guide. On subsequent sessions this time may be increased, and the activities extended using games and songs from the Halliwick method suitably modified (Reid Campion, 1985).

The mother is shown various ways of holding her baby in the water. The main positions used are vertical, supine lying and prone lying. In the vertical position support is given by the mother's hands at the upper chest or mid trunk depending on the child's head and truncal development (Fig. 10.1). In supine the mother has the child's head on her shoulder and supports the body with the hands. When the prone lying position is used the baby's upper trunk is supported by the mother's shoulder, while her hands support the child's legs (Fig. 10.2).

When the baby requires full support for the head and body he is cradled in the mother's arms as shown in Fig. 10.3. The child is facing his mother who supports the child's head with one hand and the body with the other. This is a good position to develop and enhance eye contact. This cradling can be modified as head control improves (Fig. 10.4).

From the first session onwards action songs can be initiated. These are carried out gently from the beginning but as the baby

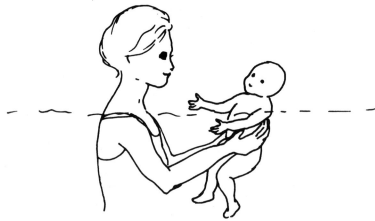

Fig. 10.1 Child with good head control

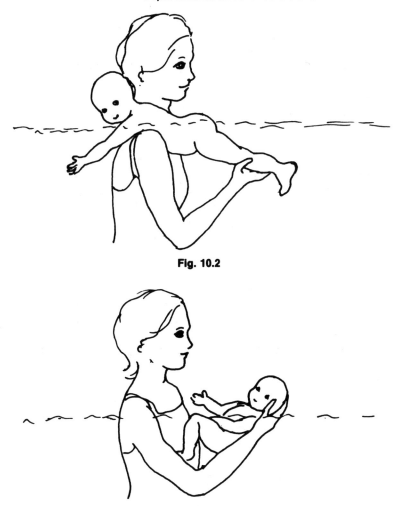

Fig. 10.2

Fig. 10.3 Full support for the head

becomes more confident they become more vigorous. If a baby is not ready to be taken through the songs even when conducted slowly and gently, he is held close as the mother moves through the water. Water toys are often floated on the surface to break up the large expanse of water; this helps to increase the baby's confidence.

Following the programme of activities for the child, the mothers leave the pool and dress first while the physiotherapist who has been in the water throughout, holds the babies in rotation handing

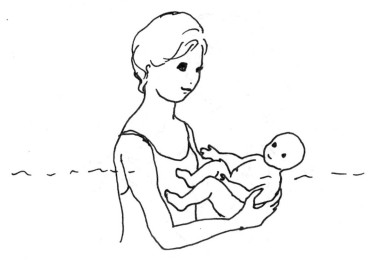

Fig. 10.4 Cradling used when there is greater head control

over the child to its mother as she leaves the changing area. Prior to leaving the department the mother should have the opportunity to feed her baby, particularly as the majority of the babies are either hungry or thirsty after the pool sessions. This is also an opportunity for the mothers to socialize and discuss with each other their children, difficulties and successes.

DEVELOPMENTAL FACTORS

Physiotherapists need to be aware of certain developmental facts so that these can be explained to the mothers when questions are raised.

Density

A comment often made is 'my baby feels as if he will float'. This phenomenon is quite normal and is due to the infant's specific density of approximately 0.86 when compared to the specific density of water.

Reflex Swimming Action

'Swimming is one of the oldest phylogenetic functions of which there is a residual in the behaviour of the newborn infant' (McGraw, 1969). The neuromuscular organization for such a pattern requires a high level of control over and above that needed for other behaviours such as creeping. McGraw (1969) suggests that when faced with more difficult and dangerous situations the infant uses subcortical centres rather than cortical areas which are less developed, to combine motor actions.

The reflex swimming action involves alternate reflex movements of the legs and arms. This takes place when an infant is immersed face down in the water and these movements may even propel the infant a little way through the water. The baby is not able to swim but the reflex movements of the arms and legs are reminiscent of a swimming action (Quinn, 1981; Reid Campion, 1985).

These swimming movements appear when the infant is exposed to water and take the form of flexion and extension of the limbs, especially the lower limbs. According to McGraw (1969) the movements range through reflex swimming to disorganized actions to voluntary movements and in the latter phase represent more automatic movements to gain a more secure environment. The acquisition of sufficient head extension above the surface to breathe comes at a later date, thus the infant's head must be supported when placed prone in the water.

This reflex has been noted as early as 11 days of age; the movements are rhythmical and usually disappear around five to six months of age (Cratty, 1979). After 8 months of age movement in the water begins to be more deliberate and kicking and cycling motions become increasingly vigorous.

The Supine Position

The child who is becoming proficient at sitting may dislike the supine position in the pool. Although this can be seen in older children, who are further advanced in their motor development it may be that the child is busily observing the environment. As a stage in development of activity in water disliking the supine position may be expected; with ingenuity and by distraction the physiotherapist can deal with this problem and it is one that usually passes quite rapidly. There have been no specific studies of the effects of relaxation classes in the hydrotherapy pool for mothers and their infants. Sweeney (1983) found that premature infants when introduced to water baths and activity was encouraged there was improvement in abnormal muscle tone, enhancement of visual and auditory orientation responses, improvement in feeding behaviour and an increase in parent participation.

Similar effects have been noted in the children who participate in the programmes offered as a postnatal service to mothers and their children in Western Australia.

This early introduction of the child to water may continue as the child develops as a water familiarization programme and form the basis of learning to swim. Children who have made friends with water at an early age are more likely to accept learning to swim more readily (Elkington, 1978). Physical activity has been shown to be vital to both normal growth of the child and to its psychological well-being (Bailey, 1976). Van Vliet and Howell (1973) state that 'there is perhaps no physical activity that can contribute to more of the combined physical, social and emotional development than swimming and diving'; it helps growth, self esteem and confidence and provides a sport that can be used from the cradle to the grave.

Swimming is a skill that has to be learnt. Early independence in water may occur in the water familiarization programme and depending on the child's physical and mental development the teaching of swimming can be gradually introduced under optimal conditions of trust and safety by a suitably trained instructor who has a sound knowledge and understanding of child development, both physical and emotional, and who values the parents' cooperation and encourages their involvement.

REFERENCES

Auckett D. A. (1981). '*Baby Massage*' Melbourne: Hill of Content.

Bailey D. A. (1976). 'The growing child & the need for physical activity'. In *Child in Sport & Physical Activity* (Albinson J. G., Andrew G. M. eds). Baltimore: University Park Press.

Barnett B., Blignaut I., Holmes S. *et al.* (1987). Quality of attachment in a sample of one year old Australian children. *Journal of American Academy of Child and Adolescent Psychiatry*, **26(3)**, 303–307.

Cobb J. (1980). *Babyshock: A mother's first five years*. London: Hutchinson.

Cratty B. J. (1979). *Perceptual and Motor Development in Infants and Children* 2nd edn., New Jersey: Prentice Hall Inc.

Elkington H. (1978). Swimming: a handbook for teachers. Cambridge: Cambridge University Press.

Euler C., Soderberg U. (1956). The relation between gamma motor activity and the electroencephalogram. *Experientia* 12, 278.

Harris R., McInnes M. (1963). Exercises in water. In *Medical Hydrology*, (Licht S. ed.) pp 207–17. New Haven: Elizabeth Licht.

Harris S. R. (1978). Neurodevelopmental treatment approach for teaching swimming to cerebral palsied children, *Physical Therapy*, 58(8), 979–983.

Kraus R. (1973). *Therapeutic Recreation Service Principles and Practices*, Philadelphia: W. B. Saunders Company.

Leboyer F. (1975). *Birth without Violence*, New York: Alfred A. Knopf.

Levine B. A. (1984). Use of hydrotherapy in reduction of anxiety, *Psychological Reports*, 55, 526.

Madders J. (1979). Stress and relaxation. Sydney: Collins.

McGraw M. B. (1969). *The Neuromuscular Maturation of the Human Infant*. New York: Hafner Publishing Company.

Mertin P. G. (1986). Maternal–infant attachment: a developmental perspective. *Australian and New Zealand Journal of Obstetrics and Gynaecology*, 26, 196–198.

Mitchell L. (1987). *Simple Relaxation: the Mitchell Method of Physiological Relaxation for Easing Tension*. 2nd edn. London: Murray.

Quinn S. (1981). *Water Babies*, Report from Northern Ireland Sports Council.

Piaget J. (1963). *The Origins of Intelligence in Children*, New York: W. W. Norton and Co. Inc.

Reid Campion M. (1985). *Hydrotherapy in Paediatrics*, Oxford: Heinemann Medical.

Shepherd R. (1980). *Physiotherapy in Paediatrics* 2nd edn. Oxford: Heinemann Medical.

Skinner A., Thomson A. (1983). *Duffield's Exercise in Water* 3rd edn., London: Ballière Tindall.

Sweeney J. K. (1983). Neonatal hydrotherapy adjunct to developmental intervention in an intensive care nursery setting. In *Aquatics: A Revived Approach to Paediatric Management*, (Dulcy F. H. ed), pp. 39–52. City Haworth Press Inc.

Van Vliet M. A., Howell M. L. (1973). *Be Water Wise*. Canada: The Canadian Red Cross Society and the Royal Life Saving Society Canada.

Whiteford B., Polden M. (1984). *Postnatal Exercises*, London: Courtesy Publishing Co. Ltd.

Wilson I. H., Kasch F. W. (1963). Medical aspects of swimming. In *Medical Hydrology* (Licht S. ed), New Haven; Elizabeth Licht, Publisher.

Water Fitness for the Older Adult

Water can be an ideal medium for conditioning exercises for the older adult. It is well documented that regular exercise can minimize the effects of biological ageing and it follows that an exercise programme would act to help older people maintain independence and mobility so that they can continue to take part in the activities they enjoy (Pardini, 1984). A water programme can be an attractive alternative even for those who do not swim. Often as confidence improves in the water, some people find that they can learn this new skill and it is a tremendous boost to their morale.

SETTING UP A WATER FITNESS PROGRAMME

In setting up a water fitness programme a number of practical considerations must be taken into account if the programme is to be effective and conducted in safety.

Facilities

The facilities must be investigated to ensure that the participants have ease of entry and exit to the pool. It would be preferable to have a ramp but if no ramp is available someone can be positioned near the steps to assist those individuals who request help. As well as entry and exit into the pool it should be remembered that the most common accidents in this age group are frequently caused by poor balance, slow recovery time after being thrown off balance, dizziness and tendency to trip over materials at the side of the pool.

Ideally hand rails need to be provided and non-slip surfaces in all areas of the pool and change rooms would lead to greater safety for the elderly.

Water Temperature

The water temperature should be between 28–32°C in winter and 1–

2° less in summer. If the water is a little cool an immediate effect could be involuntary hyperventilation and a rise in blood pressure. It must be remembered that water conducts heat away from the body much more rapidly than air. It is advisable to remind the participants to cool their skin before entering the pool and to immerse themselves gradually.

Emergency Procedure

It is essential to establish an emergency procedure and to delegate some of the responsibilities such as phoning for medical assistance to another person, leaving the class leader to deal with the immediate circumstances. The leader should have a whistle to blow to attract everyone's attention and to ensure that the participants cease their activity and remain still whilst the emergency is dealt with. Regular emergency procedure rehearsals are advantageous in ensuring the understanding and cooperation of the group participants. Any leader of a group must be competent with cardiopulmonary resuscitation (CPR) techniques.

A leader taking an exercise class for the older adults must know of any specific problems that members of the group may have, that would affect activity in an aquatic environment. Some instructional modifications may be required for instance if participants wear glasses. It is advisable to keep these on during the class as this will assist the participants to see demonstrations better. Hearing aids should not be worn in the water so if the participant has a hearing problem it is important to be paired with someone of good hearing. In presenting instructions it is prudent to understand that neural information reception and the capacity for processing are decreased with age. These instructions should be at a slow pace with concrete demonstrations (Piscopo, 1979). An increase in reaction time indicates that games involving decision making need to be played at a slower pace and rules can be modified to take this into account.

The leader should have a high profile so that she can be seen and heard at all times. It may be necessary to stand on the pool edge if the pool is particularly noisy and the class is large. It is found that between 15–18 people is a maximum number of participants in a class. Any more than this makes the class dangerous as the leader can not supervise adequately.

ADVANTAGES AND BENEFITS TO THE ELDERLY

The benefits of exercising in water are many. For those individuals with arthritic conditions there is less stress on the muscles and joints. The body weight is supported and a person immersed in water to the neck experiences about 90% of their body weight being relieved. The effect of support of body weight results in less stress on the joints and muscles themselves which in turn enables a greater range of movement at the joint. For older people with osteoporosis the water provides a very safe environment for exercising. Water also provides a medium where falls do not have the same consequences as those on dry land. Recent literature shows that water may be a medium in which the osteoporotic person may add to bone density as swimming is said to increase bone density in men and is likely to add bone density to women (Orwoll, 1987).

Shephard (1984) reports that where an older person's venous tone is poor the counterpressure of water on the legs reduces the tendency for blood to pool in the legs. This effect can be increased if the person is horizontal as in swimming. Exercising in the water can provide an excellent environment to improve endurance, cardio-vascular, cardiorespiratory and muscular activity, and it enhances strength, flexibility, balance and coordination. Importantly it is fun, refreshing and relaxing too.

PROGRAMMES

A programme format can be devised taking into consideration the specific benefits required. Assessment of participants is vital and any new member of the class should be checked before undertaking activity in the water. A medical check for blood pressure, medical problems and medications is advisable.

The leader must constantly assess to make certain that activities are progressed at an appropriate rate for all group members and it is sometimes necessary to cater for different levels of fitness within the group. Time should be spent prior to the commencement of a class in advising the group about signs of over exertion such as persistent fatigue during the following day after exercise, persistent muscular aches and pains, unusual restlessness and insomnia (Wear, 1977).

Signals for ceasing exercise are explained to the group. These include fainting, light headedness or dizziness, any chest pain referred to the arm, teeth or ear, nausea or irregular heart rate. If any of these signs are noticed it may be necessary to refer the participant to a doctor. The pool could be a new environment for some individuals and the physiotherapist should teach the techniques of mental adjustment and balance restoration (Reid Campion, 1985) to reduce tension and in the interests of safety.

Components of the Class

The components of the class are:

1. Stretching/warm-up (for stretching exercises see p. 207)
2. Aerobic activity
3. Strengthening exercises
4. Games e.g. team games
5. Cool down, include flexibility exercises, balance and coordination and slow gentle stretching (see p. 216)

1. Stretching/warm-up

In this component of the programme it is important that the heart rate is raised gradually, walking laps are used here, and all major areas of the body are stretched adequately. Advice on how to stretch would be provided especially when any new participants join the class. Such advice serves as a precautionary measure and allows reinforcement whenever a new member attends.

Exercising with a partner is an extremely useful way to increase the sociability of the group.

2. Aerobic activity

Brisk walking is an example of an aerobic activity used in the water programme and this can be sustained for 12–15 minutes.

Members of the class can start walking in deeper water and the difficulty of the activity can be progressed by walking in progressively shallower water which leads to more gravity loading on the skeleton. However, walking and any activity in deeper water, though giving increased buoyancy does demand considerably harder work in moving more of the body through the water against turbulence and demands greater balance and coordination. Difficulty can also be increased by using such walking exercises as zig-zagging, asking participants to walk in one diagonal direction for a few steps then in the opposite direction thus creating turbulence against which the person must work. Walking backwards and then forwards is another way in which participants work against their own turbulence (Williams, 1987).

Many variations can be introduced to make walking laps of the pool more interesting. Walking forwards, backwards keeping head and hands forward, striding and soldier walking using opposite arm and leg are examples.

In any group setting dancing is a useful aerobic activity and it is also fun. There are many dances from which to select a routine and some samples are given. Any dance which involves facing a partner and holding hands and alternatively flexing and extending the arms should be avoided thus preventing injury, to those participants with osteoporosis as that movement and its associated lumbar rotation can precipitate crush lumbar vertebral fractures. However, care must be taken and the participants instructed to avoid rapid movements especially spinal extension and rotation. The individual should perform these movements purposefully and with control.

3. Strengthening component

Some exercises are given later in the chapter consisting of specific exercises for various parts of the body using the water as resistance. Extra resistance can be provided where required by the use of kickboards.

4. Game component

Games are immensely popular and the ball games of over and under, and tunnel ball are great favourites. Maintaining well tuned reflexes is a primary benefit to be gained from these activities. Some examples are given later in the chapter.

5. Cool down

This segment should be gradual and can include flexibility or coordination exercises and appropriate slow stretching which may be similar to those at the start of the class.

Assessment

Every six weeks or so a 12 minute walk, jog or swim test should be given. The participants measure their pulse, a skill learnt on joining the fitness group. The pulse is taken before and after the walk, swim or jog. The number of laps are measured as a progress monitor for the participants.

It needs to be understood that work performed in water will vary directly with the projected area of the body parts and the depth of submersion. Thus, if the development of cardiorespiratory fitness is desired faster movement will produce great turbulent effect and thus increased work during exercise.

In the older group the intensity of the exercise prescriptions can be 60% of the maximum heart rate reserve. The maximum heart rate being considered to be 220 BPM – age (Gibbs, 1981). Cognizance must be given to the fact that when exercising in water or swimming 10–13 heartbeats/minute should be subtracted from the age predicted maximum (McCardle *et al.*, 1986).

If an aerobic effect is wanted the duration and frequency of exercise are important. Fifteen to twenty minutes of continuous aerobic activity three to four days a week is said to have a positive effect on fitness (Gibbs, 1981). In this case it is important for the physiotherapist to stress the need for some physical activity the members can enjoy at home as an addition to their water exercise class.

LEADERSHIP QUALITIES

The physiotherapist is well advised to have some cognizance of strategies for working with adults. It is important to remember people, their names, appearance, particular likes or dislikes of the individual. The programme could also include 'getting acquainted' activities.

At times it is appropriate to share the leadership by asking for favourite exercises or perhaps letting a class member conduct an exercise or activity. Recognition of achievement is a very positive part of group work. Everyone likes to feel their efforts and progress have been noticed. This gives reinforcement and acts as an incentive to further action (Alberta Recreation Development Division, 1978).

Adults rarely like being singled out for attention so that when an exercise or activity is being performed incorrectly suggestions as to how to improve an action should be made to the whole group. Safety measures can be built into the programmes so that a particular participant does not draw attention to himself by verbal identification of a problem or limitation, for example, loss of balance. This relatively common disability after the age of 50 can be catered for by balance activities being built into the programme.

Motivating the participants to take responsibility for monitoring their own fitness levels and being aware that it is not competitive or stressful is an important leadership strategy.

The use of music can be a motivating ingredient in a class situation. It is an extremely useful tool for encouraging interaction, increasing range of movements as well as facilitating ease of movement (Cross, 1984). Participants may even sing along with the music. Some pools, however, are very noisy and music in these circumstances may create a confusing atmosphere.

Water fitness programmes for the older citizen encourages the individual to take part in an activity which has enormous physical and mental benefits. The activity extends the participant's sphere of social contact; exercising, playing and laughing together are a firm basis on which friendships can develop. Those taking part in the fitness class affirm that they are 'adding life to years'.

STRENGTHENING EXERCISES

1. The participant is prone lying, holding the bar with one hand, the other placed lower on the wall then doing flutter kicks. This exercise can also be carried out holding onto the bar in side lying then doing side stroke kick.
2. Standing holding onto the bar with one hand sideways doing leg abduction and adduction. This exercise can also be done facing the wall and holding the bar with both hands.
3. Standing sideways, holding the bar with one hand, hip flexion and extension keeping the knee extended and the body upright.
4. Stride standing sideways, holding a kickboard below the surface of the water with two hands, push the kickboard fowards and pull it back towards the body.
5. Stride standing sideways holding the kickboard with two hands push the board down below the surface of the water and controlling its return to the surface.

GAMES

Examples of games are as follows:

1. Numbers huddle (*Life Be In It Games Manual, 1981*)—the whole group moves freely in a space designated by the leader. The leader calls a number and individuals make a group of this number. Those who do not join a group drop out. Continue until two or three people are left.

2. Whirlpool—The whole group makes one circle. The circle begins walking clockwise and leads into walking more quickly. Once a whirlpool has been created everyone submerges to shoulders and relaxes, and is carried around in the whirlpool.

3. Activities using ball (e.g. Over/under relay)—teams of equal number have a ball at the beginning of their line. On the word 'go' they pass the ball overhead and under through their legs alternatively. When the last person gets the ball they move to the beginning until everyone has had a turn.

DANCE ROUTINES

1. Allemande—partners in a circle facing each other and holding right hands, pass by the partner with the right hand and walk on to the next, grasping their left hand with your left hand and passing by. This is an excellent getting to know you activity with members greeting each other by name.

Many of the 'old time' dance steps can be carried out in the water and favourites such as the progressive barn dance are often used.

2. Hucklebuck—participants in straight lines, e.g. four abreast could be suitable depending on the width of the pool.
The routine is:

- 4 steps forward right, left right left
- 4 jumps backwards, zigzag
- 2 star jumps, out in, out in
- 2 hops left foot, lift right knee
- 2 hops right foot, lift left knee
- 1 hop left foot, lift right knee

- 1 hop right foot, lift left knee
- 1 jump feet apart quarter turn to the right.

STRETCHING

In the following exercises, the participant is standing.

1(a) With the feet spaced comfortably apart, standing sideways. Side stretch—hold one hand above head, bend sideways carrying the arm over the head. Hold for 3 seconds and return to the starting position. If necessary for stability, the participant can hold the bar with the other hand and stretch sideways and forwards to the side of the pool.

 (b) Shoulder stretch—extend straight arms behind the body. Hold for 3 seconds.

 (c) Hamstring stretch—bring one knee towards chest and hold against chest with one or both hands for 3 seconds.

 (d) A lunge standing sideways, adductor stretch—place one leg out sideways with the knee flexed and take the body weight forwards and sideways onto that foot. Push slowly over bent knee and foot. Hold for 3 seconds.

 (e) With the feet comfortably apart, turn the trunk first to one side then to the other.

 (f) Quadriceps stretch—bend one leg up behind and hold the foot with one hand, the other hand may be needed to support yourself by holding the bar, pull the foot upwards so that you can feel the thigh muscle being stretched. Hold for 3 seconds.

 (g) Lunge standing forwards, calf stretch—lean forward on to one leg with forward knee bent. Push slowly forward keeping back heel on ground. Hold for 3 seconds.

Diagrams of many of these stretches are included in the chapter on Hydrotherapy in the Childbearing Year.

SUMMARY

A format for a water fitness class for the older adult has been presented. Important considerations in setting up such a class and the necessary precautions are discussed. The value of this form of exercise for this age group cannot be doubted; the comments and obvious enjoyment of the participants speak for themselves.

REFERENCES

Alberta Recreation Development Division Senior Citizens Sports and Games Manual (1978), Alberta: Alberta Recreation Development Division.

Cooper C. Y. (1976). Swimming for senior citizens, *Therapeutic Recreation Journal*, **2**, 50–54.

Cross P., McHellenan M., Vomberge Mowga T. W. (1984). Observations on the use of music in the rehabilitation of stroke patients, *Physiotherapy* (Canada) **34**, 197–201.

Gibbs R. (1981). *Exercise for the Over 50's*, Victoria: Sun Books Pty Ltd.

Harrison R., Bulstrode F. (1987). Percentage weight bearing during partial immersion in the hydrotherapy pool, *Physiotherapy Practice*, **13**(2), 60–63.

McArdle W. D., Katch F. I., Katch V. L. (1981). *Exercise Physiology — Energy, Nutrition and Human Performance*, Philadelphia: Lea and Febiger.

Life Be In It Games Manual (1981), Victoria. Sun Books Pty Ltd

Orwoll E. S., Ferar, J. L., Oviatt S. K., et al. (1987) The effect of swimming exercise on bone mineral content, *Abstract Clin. Res.* **35**(1), 194A.

Pardini A. (1984). Exercise, vitality and aging, *Aging*, **344**, 19–29.

Piscopo J. (1979). Indications and contraindications of exercise and activity for older persons. *Journal of Physical Education & Recreation*. **50**(9), 31–34.

Reid Campion M. (1985). *Hydrotherapy in Paediatrics*, Oxford: Heinemann Medical.

Shephard, R. J. (1984) 'Physical activity for seniors, a role for pool exercises: *Canadian Association for Health Physical Education & Recreation* **50**(6), 2–5, 20.

Wear, R. G., (1977). Conditioning exercise programme for normal older persons. In *Guide to Fitness after 50*. (Harris, R. and Frankel, J.) New York: Plenum Press.

Index

Achilles tendonitis 186–7
acromioclavicular joint
    injuries 182–5
allemande 243
ankle, ligamentous injuries 185–6
ankylosing spondylitis 144–7
  aims of treatment 144
  free exercise programme 145
  hold-relax techniques 127
  posture check 147
  swimming 146, 147
  techniques 144–5
    stretching 146–7
aqua-aerobics 176
Aqua-Ark 192
aqua-relaxation,
    mother/child 224–34
  aims 224–5
  anxiety reduction 225–6
  assessment 228–9
  baby's density 232
  criteria 227–8
  head control 226, 230–2
  procedure 229–32
  referrals 228
  reflex swimming action 233
  relaxation 225
  righting reactions,
    head/truncal 226
  self support 226
  sensory-motor
    development 226–7
  supine position 233–4
assessment 13–14
ataxia:
  cerebellar 95
  sensory 95–6

back pain 142–3
Bad Ragaz patterns 12, 23–5
  ligamentous knee injuries 182
  orthopaedic conditions 159
  rheumatoid arthritis 127
  spinal injuries 188
  stress fractures 179
  unsuitability for groupwork 32
balance exercises 98
balance reaction re-education 79–80
balance restoration 18–19
  lateral rotation 18–19
  vertical rotation 18
Baruch, Dr. Simon 5
base of skull fracture 66
Bernoulli's theorem 7
body shape/density analysis 16–17
Braxton Hicks contractions 204
breathing exercises 85–6
  breath control 86
  in water 25
  lateral thoracic expansion 86–7
buoyancy 21, 73

cauda equina lesions 117
cerebellum 48
  damage effect on tonus 51
cervical spine rotation 28
childbearing year see pregnant
    woman
cohesion 21
contracture reduction 75–6
Crohn's disease arthritis 143

degenerative arthritis 140; see also
    osteoarthritis

disc degeneration 140
dyspraxic patient 60

elbow:
    arthroplasty 174
    fractures 174
equilibrium reaction
        re-education 79–80, 98
exercise in water 22–31
    Bad Ragaz patterns *see* Bad
        Ragaz patterns
    body rotating 28
    body shapes changing 27
    body tilting 28
    breathing exercises 25
    buoyancy assisted, supported,
        resisted 23
    hold-relax techniques 25
    repeated contractions 25
    stabilization 25
    static muscle work 29–31
    techniques using
        buoyancy/balance 26
    using turbulence 26, 28–9

Fembrace 203
femur:
    fractured neck 162–3
    fractured shaft 166–7
    slipped upper epiphysis 165–6
    supracondylar fracture 169
fibromyalgia 148
fibrositis 148–52
    clinical symptoms 148
    tender/trigger points 148
    treatment 148–52
fibula, fractured 180–1
Floyer, Sir John 4, 39
friction 8, 21
Froude (1810–79) 8

gait retraining 29
    lower motor neuron/spinal cord
        lesions 83–4
    spinal cord injuries 83–4
    upper motor neuron lesions 84–5

gait, 'robot' walking pattern 56
Girdlestone arthroplasty 164
glenohumeral joint dislocation 183
goniometry 157
'goose-step' 29
Greek hydrotherapy 4, 39
group work 31–2
Guillain-Barré syndrome 72–3
    balance/equilibrium reaction
        re-education 79–80
    hip adductor stretch 73–4
    muscle strengthening 76

hamstring stretches 74–5
hemiplegic arm stretches 74
hip:
    Girdlestone arthroplasty 164–5
    total replacement 163
hip adductor stretch 73–4
Hippocrates (c. 460–375 BC) 39
historical background 3–5
hold-relax techniques 25, 127
Hubbard tank 5, 21
huckleback 243
humerus:
    fractured neck 172–3
    fractured shaft 174
hydrodynamical principles 6–9
    friction 8, 21
    hydrostatic pressure 8–9
    metacentre 7–8
    relative density 6
    turbulence 7, 21
hydrogymnastics 21
hydrostatic pressure 8–9
hypertonia 71
hypothalamus 9
hypotomia 71

impedance 22
inflammatory arthritis *see*
        rheumatoid arthritis

knee:
    ligamentous injuries 180–2
    reconstruction of soft tissue 168
    total replacement 167–8

knee flexion in standing 90–1
Kniepp, Sebastian 5

lateral rotation 18–19
legs, extensor group
    strengthening 97–8
lemniscal tract 47
low back pain, lateral rotation
    in 19
lower motor neuron lesion, gait
    retraining 83–4

mental adjustment 17–18
metacentre 7–8
motor pattern re-education 77
movement retraining 89–90
multiple sclerosis 100, 101–2
multisystems degeneration 96
muscle spindle 43, 44
muscle strengthening 76
muscle stretching 72–3
muscle tone:
    heat effects on 43
    reduction by vestibular
        stimulation 44–5

neck exteroceptors 43
neurological conditions:
    curled up (ball) position 28
    gait retraining 29
    hydrotherapy effects 11
neurological rehabilitation 70–102
    adverse reactions to
        hydrotherapy 100–2
    clinical aims 71–2
        contracture prevention 72–3
        increased/decreased muscle
            tone 71–2
    contraindications to
        hydrotherapy 99–100
    fitness/psychological effects 87–9
    indications for hydrotherapy 71
    movement retraining 89–90
neuro-surgical patient 41–68
    hydrotherapy 43–66
        access functional movement
        patterns 60–3
        breath control development 63
        cardio-vascular fitness
            increase 65
        centralized (rotational) pattern
            of movement retraining 56
        contra-indications 66–7
        movement stimulating 47–50
        orthopaedic complications 64
        psychological effects 63–4
        reciprocal pattern movement
            retraining 58–9
        recreation/socialization 65–6
        righting reactions
            retraining/stimulation 51–4
        tone decreasing 43–6
        untoward effects 67
        voice production 63
        weak movements
            augmenting/range
            increasing 55–6

O'Donoghue triad 181
oedematous limbs 64
older adult, water fitness 236–44
    advantages/benefits 238
    aerobic activity 239–40
    assessment 241
    dance routines 243
    emergency procedure 237
    facilities 236
    games 243
    leader 237
    leadership qualities 241–2
    programmes 238–40
    strengthening exercises 240, 242
    stretching exercises 244
    water temperature 237
orthopaedic conditions 155–75
    assessment 157
    Bad Ragaz techniques 159
    classwork 157
    exercise progression 159–61
    signs and symptoms 155–6
    swimming 156, 158 (table)

*see also specific orthopaedic
   conditions*
osteoarthrosis 140
   spinal 142
   treatment 140–1
   precautions 124
Owata Obi 203

paraplegia 116–17
   hydrotherapy 116–17
   innervation levels 118 (table)
Parkinson's disease 96–7, 98
Pascal's law 8
patella, fractured 169
percentage weight-bearing in
   water 156
physiotherapist's presence in
   pool 12–13, 22
Piaget's theory of
   development 226–7
polystyrene, submersion
   pressure 128
postnatal exercise class 219
postnatal swimming 222
pregnant woman 199–222
   aerobics 209–12
   Braxton Hicks contractions 204
   breathing exercises 216–17
   calf-stretch 207
   contraindicated water sports 222
   depth of water 205
   exercise classes 199
   hamstring stretch 207
   ligament softening 203
   music for exercising 220
   physical benefits of exercising in
      water 201–3
   postnatal exercise class 219
   quadriceps stretch 207
   rotation stretch 208–9
   screening/safety 204–5
   shoulder stretches 204
   side lunge 208
   strengthening exercises 212–16
   swimming 220–2
      postnatal 222

twelve minute walk test 201
water fitness class 200–1, 205–6
   warm up 206
water fitness programmes 203–4
water temperature 205
Pressnitz, Vincent 5
proprioceptive neuromuscular
   facilitation techniques 48–50
psoriatic arthritis 144
pubic rami fracture 162

radius, fractured 174–5
recording of
   assessment/treatment 14–16
re-education of motor patterns 77
Reiter's disease 144
relative density 6
resistance:
   on land 22
   water 21
reticular formation 47, 48
rheumatic disease 123–47
   aims of treatment 124–5
   assessment/planning of
      treatment 123
   clinical signs/symptoms 123
   hydrotherapy
      contra-indications 123–4
   see also rheumatoid arthritis
rheumatoid arthritis 125–39
   aims of treatment 125
   education of patient 129–30
   elbow arthroplasty 174
   entry into pool 126–7
   exercises 130, 131–2
   functional activities 135
   group treatments 128–9, 132
   hold-relax techniques 127
   individual programme 126
   mobility programme 132–5
   mobilization 127
   muscle strengthening 127–8
   post-therapy treatment 139
   posture 133–4
   procedure prior to exercise
      programme 125–6

rheumatoid arthritis—*cont.*
  relaxation 131, 136
  safety procedures 126, 136–9
  swimming 136
  treatment time 139
  water temperature 125
rolling in the horizontal 78–9
Roman hydrotherapy 4, 39
rotation:
  lateral 18–19
  vertical 18
rotator cuff impingement
    syndrome 183
running in water 192–4

sensorimotor development 226
sensory ataxia 95–6
sero-negative spondarthritis
    (spondyloarthropathies) 144;
    see also ankylosing spondylitis
Shaw, Dr. Joel 5
shoulder:
  abduction 94
  capsulitis 92, 93–4
  flexion 94
  horizontal abduction 91
  horizontal
    abduction-adduction 95
  pain, swiming-induced 183
  painful hemiplegic 92
  tendonitis 92, 93–4
shoulder arthroplasty 173–4
shoulder girdle:
  sports injuries 182–5
  tone reduction 88–9
shoulder-hand syndrome 92, 92–3
sitting balance exercise 80–1
sitting or standing balance
    exercise 82–3
SOAP assessment 14
SOAPIER assessment 14–15
spasticity, reduction by rotation
    around longitudinal axis of
    body 45
speech pathologist (therapist) 63

spinal cord injuries, hydrotherapy
    for 104–21
  advantages 104–5
  aims of treatment 107–10
    neurologically impaired
      patient 107–9
    neurologically intact
      patient 110
  disadvantages 105–7
  ear problems 106–7
  entering/leaving pool 120–1
  hydrotherapy
      techniques 110–21
    cauda equina lesions 117
    exercise 114
    high cervical   lesions 111–12
    incomplete paraplegic
      patient 117
    incomplete tetraplegic
      patient 116
    low cervical lesions 112
    mid cervical lesions 112
    neurologically impaired
    patient 110–19
    neurologically intact
    patient 119–21
    paraplegic patient 116–17
    recreation 118–19
    swimming 114–16
  incontinent patient 106
  precautions 105–7
  respiratory distress 105
  temperature regulation 106
spinal cord injuries, gait
    retraining 83–4
spondyloarthropathies
    (sero-negative
    spondarthritis) 143; *see also*
    ankylosing spondylitis
spine, sports injuries 187–8
spinothalamic tract 47
sports injuries 176–94
  classification 177
  hydrotherapy treated 177–8
  programme organisation 189–91

rehabilitation principles 188–9
running in water 192–4
see also specific injuries
standing balance exercise 81–2
standing to lying to standing
  through sitting 77–8
static muscle work 29–31
sternoclavicular joint injuries 182–5
stress fractures 178
stroke 87–8
supranuclear palsy 96
suture lines 158
swimming 33–6
  ankylosing spondylitis
    patient 146, 147
  balance restoration 36
  breathing control 36
  fractured radius/ulna 175
  Halliwick method 33
  mental adjustment 35
  neonatal reflex action 233
  orthopaedic patient 157, 158
    (table)
  osteoporotic patient 143
  postnatal 222
  pregnant woman 220–2
  rheumatoid arthritis patient 136
  Roman exercise 39
  shoulder pain in competitive
    swimmers 183
  spinal cord lesions 114–16
  stroke selection 34–5

temperature, body 9
tetraplegia:
  hydrotherapy 112–13, 116
  innervation levels 111 (table)
thalamus 48
thermal information carriage in
  neural pathways 47–8

thermoregulatory system 9
  neuro-surgical patient 43–4
tibia:
  fractured 170–1
  osteotomy 170
  plateau fracture 169
tibialis posterior transfer 171–2
triple pelvic osteotomy 161–2
trunk:
  extensor group
    strengthening 97–8
  rotation exercise 97
  tone reduction 88–9
turbulence 7, 21, 27
  use of 28–9
turning in the vertical 78
twelve minute walk test 201

ulcerative colitis, arthritic 144
ulna, fractured 174–5

vertical rotation 18
vestibular-occular reflex 48
vestibular stimulation 44, 48
viscosity 21

water:
  bow wave effect 22, 24
  drag wave effect 24
  energy expended while exercising
    in 202
  exercise in *see* exercise in water
    resistance 21
  temperature of exercise 9–12
Wesley, John 4–5, 39
Wetvests 119
Winterwitz, Professor 5
Wright, Dr 5

Zahm (1862–1945) 8